AREQUIPA SANATORIUM

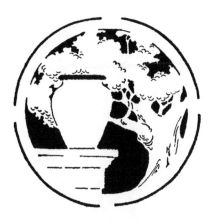

AREQUIPA
SANATORIUM

LIFE IN CALIFORNIA'S
LUNG RESORT FOR WOMEN

~

LYNN DOWNEY

UNIVERSITY OF OKLAHOMA PRESS : NORMAN

Publication of this book is made possible through the generosity of Edith Kinney Gaylord.

LIBRARY OF CONGRESS CATALOGING-IN-PUBLICATION DATA

Names: Downey, Lynn, 1954– author.
Title: Arequipa Sanatorium : life in California's lung resort for women / Lynn Downey.
Description: Norman : University of Oklahoma Press, [2019] | Includes bibliographical references and index.
Identifiers: LCCN 2019001715 | ISBN 978-0-8061-6395-6 (pbk. : alk. paper)
Subjects: | MESH: Arequipa Sanatorium. | Hospitals, Chronic Disease—history | Tuberculosis, Pulmonary—history | Women—history | History, 20th Century | California
Classification: LCC RA981.C3 | NLM WF 28 AC2 | DDC 362.1109794—dc23
LC record available at https://lccn.loc.gov/2019001715

For Grandma, who started it all.
LOIS MAY BONSEY DOWNEY
1904–2006

CONTENTS

ILLUSTRATIONS

ACKNOWLEDGMENTS

Historians rely on people in the present day to write books about the past. A magnificent cheering section of friends and colleagues spurred me on as I researched and wrote this historical and yet very personal project.

During the thirty-five years I thought about writing this book, my oldest and best friend, Kay McDonough, a documentary filmmaker, urged me to focus on the people and not the place and to make my grandmother's story its center. It took me a long time to realize she was right, and I lost her to cancer before the writing was done. But Kay lived long enough to know that her wisdom gave my book its heart.

Happy and Cari Lyn Stanton not only preserved Arequipa's historical records; they became my dearest friends. I am especially grateful to Cari Lyn for sharing her Arequipa story with me.

Dr. Robert J. Chandler, the expert on all things San Francisco and frontiers beyond, had my back throughout this whole process, even before I started writing.

In addition to friendship and fabulous meals, Joe Taylor and Sheila Menzies of the Tile Heritage Foundation gave me the necessary grounding on the history of American tile and ceramics.

Waverly Lowell provided historical counsel as I learned about Arequipa's history and its archives, and was a very welcome companion on my first visit to the site (post–Girl Scouts).

Many thanks go out to my early readers for their discerning feedback on the manuscript: Dr. Robert Chandler, Patti Elkin, Jennifer Gunn, and Cari Lyn Stanton.

After I finished writing this book, but before I found the University of Oklahoma Press, members of the Brown family found me. I am deeply grateful to the many generations of Browns (and their loved ones) who shared stories, photos, meals, their homes, and their hearts with me: Sarah Brown and Alan Gourley, Andrew Brown and Olga Pang Stein, Charlotte Brown, Margot Siepelt, and Alyson Fox. They also made it possible for me to meet and spend a wonderful week with Rose Wong Tom, a former Arequipa patient who miraculously came into my life at the same time, thanks to Dr. Mike Thompson. And much gratitude to

Carole Chu and Maura Johnston for sharing your Auntie Rose with me.

I was lucky to work with a wonderful collection of librarians, archivists, and historians as I walked the writing road: Amy Catania, Mary Hotaling, and Marc Wanner of Historic Saranac Lake; Michael M. Lange of the Bancroft Library; Laurie Thompson and Carol Acquaviva of the Anne T. Kent California Room, Marin County Library; Susan Goldstein of the San Francisco History Center, San Francisco Public Library; Jean Shulman of the American Red Cross; Nathaniel Ball of Elmira College; Janet Olson of Northwestern University; Nora Murphy of the Massachusetts Institute of Technology; Jenny Johnson of Stanford University; Derek Anderson and Alexandria Brown of Marin Academy; Greg Morrison of the American Society of Radiologic Technologists; Tom Schmidt of the Sharlot Hall Museum; Frances Kaplan and Debra Kaufman of the California Historical Society; Russell Johnson and Teresa Johnson of History and Special Collections for the Sciences at the Louise M. Darling Biomedical Library at the University of California–Los Angeles, which awarded me a Charles Donald O'Malley Research Fellowship.

Jill Hunting, Steve Graydon, and Vivian Russell provided writing advice, graphics and marketing advice, good fellowship, and more great meals.

Jack Schaeffer of Act 3 Partners did his digital magic and made all my photographs shine.

All authors should have an editor as wonderful as Chuck Rankin. He championed both me and my story, and this book would not be in your hands without him. I am also grateful to Peg Goldstein for her thoughtful copyediting. And finally, many thanks to the University of Oklahoma Press for accepting me into its award-winning ranks.

I am deeply grateful as well to the women who gave me their time and their stories in my early years of Arequipa research: Phoebe Hearst Brown, Lois McMurdo, Marion Dickey, "Patty" and "Bonnie."

Many members of my large and loving family knew my grandmother and buoyed me for the decades I've thought about this project. Not all of them are still with us, but everyone is a part of this story: Mom and Dad, Jan and Doug, Papa, Jen, Ivar, Gene, Lorraine, Auntie Kee, Uncle Buck, Alton and Velma, Kathie, Mark, Cheryl, Nick, Lester, Lil, Sandy, Mark, Lisa, Phyllis, Bliss, Blissy, Brook, Marlene, Beau, myriad Ammanns, Karen, Jim, Kathleen, Pete, Terri, Paul, Patti, Julie.

And finally, all my love and thanks to Grandma, Lois May Bonsey Downey, for her courage and her willingness to let me tell her story. You made me a writer, and I miss you every day.

AREQUIPA SANATORIUM

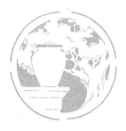

INTRODUCTION
A Memoir

THE SHARP SCENTS OF NATIVE BAY and oak hung in the air as I scrambled off the passenger seat of my mother's beige Renault and into the summer morning. The Girl Scout outing at Arequipa Day Camp in Fairfax was about to start. I waved to my mom and hurried up a long driveway that spilled into a sunlit clearing. My fellow Scouts and the adult leaders were gathered at its edge, near a rambling, brown-shingled building. Shabby looking but sturdy, it was two stories tall, with spacious, open porches.

Before setting off on a long hike, we were allowed to wander inside the place for a while. Most of the girls bolted through the open door, but I strolled in, taking my time to look around. I turned a corner and entered a dark, wood-paneled room with a large fireplace, scuffed wooden floors, and French doors made with dusty, wavy glass. I pushed these open and went down some steps onto a tiled patio that partially disappeared underneath an enormous hydrangea bush. My Keds made no noise as I walked on the neutral-colored tiles, which were a bit chipped but still in good shape. Drawn by dappled sunlight, I went back inside and found another long room with high ceilings and partially screened walls that looked out onto the porches I'd seen when I was outside. In a small nearby anteroom, I saw a metal door set up high like a wall oven, fronted with a chrome crank wheel and glass-covered dials.

I was already a confirmed history buff, and thanks to family visits to historic sites and lots of Laura Ingalls Wilder books, I was sure the building was old. I wondered what its purpose had been before legions of shouting Scouts began to cram its halls. I liked the feel of the place and started to fall under its spell, until I heard a conversation between a few other girls who had scooted into the little room behind me.

"This was a crazy house, you know," said one.

"Oh, it was not," said another.

"Yes, it was. My brother told me. Lots of nutty people lived here. And this was where they put the really bad ones." She pointed to the door with the dials.

Ten can be a gullible age, and I was very much a ten-year-old. A nuthouse it must have been. But I wasn't happy about it. The building didn't feel scary to me, just old and a bit sad. I went home and then forgot about it.

At family gatherings during these Scouting years, my paternal grandmother, Lois Downey, would sometimes start sentences with "When I was in the sanatorium . . ." This would be followed by a short monologue involving a doctor or "one of the Irish girls" or how cold the place was during the winter. I didn't ask her to elaborate, because the stories were interesting on their own. But she stopped bringing the subject up just as I got into my teen years and fell more in love with history.

I had always lived in the past, even in our brand-new housing development in Marinwood, north of San Francisco. I spent after-school hours in the fall of fifth grade on the redwood deck of my suburban home dressed in a white blouse and a long flowered skirt that my mom had made for me. There, I swept my backwoods cabin just like the mother in the TV series *Daniel Boone.*

The following spring, Mrs. Gurin taught our class about New England Puritan life by taking us into the grassy ball field behind the school buildings. She divided us into families, and we set up pretend dwellings among the native oaks that dotted the edge of the field. This was our little village of Sudbury, and we put our Puritan lessons into practice a few days a week. I loved it, but as the grass began to go brown in May, my hay fever took hold and I had to stay home the entire month. To explain my absence, my classmates said I'd been burned as a witch.

By high school I was reading fat history books and lightweight fiction set in various time periods. In 1970, during my junior year, the calico dress and granny glasses look was very popular. (Today we call it boho.) I thought this was a historical rather than a hippie look, and I decided to get one of the ruffle-fronted dresses for myself. On the first day I wore my new finery, I went into the girls' bathroom between morning classes. As I looked absently into the mirror, something clicked in my brain. With horror and a blush of shame, I realized that my button-up-the-back cotton dress was actually a nightgown.

Despite these hiccups, I stuck with history, earned a BA at San Francisco State University, and by the early 1980s was planning to attend graduate school at the University of California–Berkeley to become an archivist. History in books was one thing, but handling artifacts from the past, such as letters, photographs, quilts, dishes, and tools, had become my passion. Then, when the deadly lung disease tuberculosis reemerged in the wake of the AIDS crisis, my grandmother Lois started talking about "the sanatorium" again. One autumn day in 1983 I was visiting her in the tiny apartment she rented near the central plaza in Sonoma, about forty-five minutes from my house in Fairfax. She mentioned it again, and this time I asked her what she meant.

"What was the sanatorium?" I asked. "Why were you there?"

"Well, I had TB, dear. Tuberculosis. Dr. Philip King Brown sent me to his place called Arequipa, and that's where I got well."

"Wait a minute. Arequipa? The Girl Scout camp? The one that's a couple of miles from my house?"

"Yes, I remember the Girls Scouts took it over when it closed in . . . oh, I think it was late in the fifties sometime."

"When were you in there?"

"Well, let's see. Your father was two years old, and I went in there in November . . . it was November of 1927. I remember now."

I tried to corral the questions now crowding my brain.

"You had TB? When Daddy was a little boy? How long were you there?"

"My doctor said I only had a few months to live, so Dr. Philip King Brown let me go into Arequipa. I was there for fourteen months. I lay in bed for fourteen months and got better."

"From lying in bed?"

"That's how they cured TB back then. You just had to lie still, eat a lot of food, and breathe fresh air."

"There was a big shingled building on the property when I was there in 1965. Was that where you were?"

"That was the sanatorium, with the big wards, where my bed was. Dr. Philip King Brown built it for the working girls of San Francisco."

I was floored. I had been in the very building where my grandmother had lived for nearly two years, and it was not a loony bin. I peppered Lois with more questions and learned a number of things, including the real function of the mysterious metal door. What looked like the opening to a horror movie torture chamber was simply the door to the autoclave: where the doctors sterilized their instruments.

That was it. I had to know more about Arequipa. I went over to the Bancroft Library at the University of California–Berkeley and looked it up in the card catalog (this being the pre-internet era), but I was rewarded with only a couple of annual reports. These turned out to be pretty useful. What my grandmother had said about the place being for "working girls" was true; this Dr. Brown had built Arequipa for women who labored in factories, schools, and shops. The reports also listed the names of Arequipa's founders, how and when the sanatorium was built, and an interesting tidbit about patients making pottery for occupational therapy before World War I. Then I sat down with my grandmother in my living room and tape-recorded two hours' worth of questions.

Before we started, she opened her purse and took out a small black-and-white photograph, which she handed to me with a smile, saying, "This was taken just a few weeks before I went home." A young, smiling Lois, with a flapper haircut and dressed in an embroidered robe and slippers, posed on tiled steps beside a hydrangea covered with blooms. The joy on her face lit up the photo. Startled, I recognized the steps and the flowered bush from my long-ago Girl Scout visit.

Our interview filled a lot of holes in her personal story. My research, however, stopped dead. There was nothing in any library within driving distance. Then I got a break. I was working at the California Historical Society in San Francisco at the time, and the manuscripts curator, Waverly Lowell, listened to my tale of woe. She suggested that since the property was owned by the Girl Scouts, some historical records might have come along with it. I phoned the Northern California Girl Scout Council, and a secretary gave me the name of the site ranger out at Arequipa.

"Happy" Stanton was in charge of the Bothin Youth Center, a large tract of land that included the grounds of the old sanatorium. I called, introduced myself, and told him what I was doing. He said that when he first arrived, he found old papers and photographs scattered around the building in closets, drawers, and cupboards. The Girl Scouts told him he could just throw it all away.

My heart sank toward my shoes, but just before it hit bottom, Happy said, "I thought the stuff looked official and important. I decided to keep everything in case someone ever needed to look at it, so I boxed it up and put it in one of the sheds." When I was finally able to speak again, I made an appointment to meet him at Arequipa and asked Waverly to come with me.

I couldn't stop smiling as we drove up the driveway to the clearing I had last seen nearly twenty years before. Happy, as cheerful and enthusiastic as his name, with a strong resemblance to the young Jack London, took us directly to the shed once we had greeted each other. As trained archivists and historians, Waverly and I knew what we were looking at as soon as he opened the door.

History can pivot on the actions of just one person.

When Happy Stanton decided to keep old documents and snapshots that most people would consider trash, he ended up saving the entire forty-six-year archive of the Arequipa Sanatorium.

It was treasure. One box had nothing but photographs. Others had letters, annual reports, hand-typed newsletters, medical records, scrapbooks, and poetry. Waverly and I looked through the boxes for about a half hour, and then Happy showed us through the building. Some of the former wards were empty, while others were filled with old furniture and canoes. He also showed us a concrete bench set into the ground a few yards from the sanatorium building. Carved into its back was the name Philip King Brown, and underneath was an orange-and-blue-tiled representation of a caduceus, the ancient emblem of the doctor. Below the tile was another carving: "Founder of Arequipa." We walked around some more and thanked Happy effusively when we left. As soon as I got home, I called my grandmother to tell her about my day.

A few weeks later, I brought her back to Arequipa. She walked through the building without hesitation and into the ward where she'd spent those fourteen months. "Here's where my bed was," she said, pointing to a collection of broken bed frames near a doorway. Her smile was wide as we continued our tour.

A few years later I convinced the Girl Scouts that the materials in the shed were historically important and helped them donate everything to the Bancroft Library. I spread my net a bit wider to find more information about Arequipa, and I began to read about tuberculosis and the history of American sanatoria in general. I discovered that Arequipa was a rarity: a sanatorium created just for women.

∾

I continued to research Arequipa's history over the next decade. I found other former patients, who were happy to let me record their stories on tape. I published articles in historical journals and local newspapers, and gave lectures about the sanatorium's history around the Bay Area. In 1989 I was hired as the first in-house historian for Levi Strauss & Co. in San Francisco, and my focus as a researcher and writer shifted from TB to denim. I traveled the globe in the course of my career and shared these adventures with my grandmother, who had always wanted to see the world but never got the chance.

In the fall of 2006 I had to put my writing aside. My husband was dying of cancer, and in his last few months, my focus was on his care alone. Sleep was something I grabbed whenever I could, because I was always on alert to see if he needed anything during the night. In late September I managed to catch a short afternoon nap and slept deeply enough to have an unusual dream: I was standing by the southern end of the rainbow-decorated Robin Williams Tunnel, which links Marin County with the approach to the Golden Gate Bridge on Highway 101. Normally it swarms with cars and trucks, but in my dream the road was empty. To my right, on the western hillside, were some enormous boulders. Four women stepped out from behind them, stopped, and looked at me intently. They were dressed in the long black skirts and white blouses of the 1910s, their hair piled on their heads. With the intuition that we sometimes get in dreams, I knew they had come there from Arequipa. They began to speak, each in turn, pleading, and they all said the same thing.

"Please tell our story."

I woke up with tears on my face, consumed with an emotion that was different from the daily pain of my husband's illness. I had been thinking about Arequipa lately because my grandmother was now living in a nursing home, and watching her decline was equally painful, though it did have its moments of grace.

The intensity of the dream stayed with me for a long time but was lost in the turmoil of my husband's death in November. I moved to a smaller home a few weeks later, and as I was still unpacking, I got a phone call.

My grandmother had died in her sleep.

She was 102 years old.

As my sister, Jan, and I planned her funeral, I thought about the terror she must have felt on that long-ago day when she got her diagnosis. TB was crowding her lungs, and her own doctor gave her just months to live. So she turned to Dr. Philip King Brown. He gave her a bed, affordable treatment, and seventy-seven more years of life.

I retired from my corporate job in 2014 and began a new career as an archival consultant and writer. I wanted to take up Arequipa again and write a book about the place, and I now had the freedom to do it, though I wasn't sure where to start. So I reread the articles I'd published decades earlier.

I didn't like them very much.

They were all right as introductions to the topic, but they were impersonal and cerebral. They were more about the place than the people. They lacked emotion and sounded like undergraduate term papers. I didn't know where to go from there, but my best friend, filmmaker Kay McDonough, did. She told me there was something missing from everything I'd written: my grandmother and all the other women Arequipa was built for.

There were so many. The working women that Dr. Brown worried about. The society ladies who gave the money to build the sanatorium. The women doctors who volunteered their time and skill in a remote corner of California. The nurses who lived on the property and risked their own health to take care of the sick. The young women who started their careers as social workers. And the patients who walked with fear and weariness through Arequipa's doors.

In her book *Soul at the White Heat*, Joyce Carol Oates talks about the many motivations that inspire writers to put words on a page. One of them is "bearing witness": the obligation to give a voice to those who cannot or could not speak for themselves. The women of Arequipa had been mostly lost to time. My grandmother talked about Arequipa her whole life but didn't have the desire or skill to put pen to page. So, from the moment I interviewed her, that became my job. I didn't know then that this job would enrich my life as much as Arequipa had enriched hers.

Arequipa Sanatorium is for my grandmother, and for the man who saved her. But it is also for the others: the women she shared a ward with, the ones who cared for her, the ones she never knew but who made Arequipa possible, the survivors who gave me their stories, and the ones who met me in dreams.

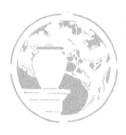

PROLOGUE
Little Girl from the Prairie

LOIS BONSEY WAS PRAIRIE-BORN and proud of it. Forest City, South Dakota, was her little village on the Missouri River, and the family lived in a part-sod house; they had to whack at the snakes that burrowed through the ceiling now and then. She grew up playing along the river's sandy banks, watching the paddle wheelers, and clumping along the wooden sidewalks in town.

Her older brother, Virgil, was a daredevil. The Missouri was his playground, and he often pulled little Lois into its temptations. Her grandparents had a store on the Cheyenne River Sioux Reservation, across the water, and Native people sometimes took the ferry that went back and forth between the two worlds to visit her father, Lewis, though this always frightened her timid mother, Mabelle.

Lewis ran a restaurant in town, and as a toddler, Lois once wandered away from the bustling café when she heard music coming from the lobby of the hotel next door. When her frantic mother found her, she was sitting on top of a piano singing along with a cowboy who was plinking out the popular song "Silver Bell." In 1908 the Bonseys welcomed another girl, named Frances, soon known as Fanny.

It was an idyllic childhood that she later compared to the novels of Mark Twain, but when she was in grammar school, the shadow of illness entered the Bonsey home. Her father lost his restaurant to an unscrupulous partner and the strain gave him a "brain fever." The family didn't know that it was really the neurological disease narcolepsy. Lewis sometimes fell asleep at the dinner table between bites or even in the middle of conversations. His doctor told him to go west or he would die. So, in early 1912, Lewis took the train to Reno, where he worked with his father, who was a cook and night watchman. Lewis toiled for six months to make enough money to bring his family to Reno. After that they planned to move to southeastern Oregon to be near relatives who ranched and raised grapes and other fruits. By the summer of 1912, a pregnant Mabelle had sewn enough clothing for herself and her three children, and they took the westward railroad, almost leaving Virgil behind at the station in Cheyenne when he got off the train to buy coffee. Reunited in Reno, the Bonseys took one more rail journey and ended up in New Pine Creek, Oregon, where Lewis worked in a grain mill and later as an agent for the Nevada-California-Oregon Railroad.

Lois and her siblings went to school, fed the chickens, and rode horses in the tree-filled landscape, so different from the prairie. Horrors still lurked though. When she was thirteen, a cousin cut off one of his toes with an ax so that he wouldn't be drafted and sent to France when the United States entered World War I. And when she was sixteen, Lois had to fend off the unwanted attentions of what can only be called a stalker, at one point hiding in the clothes hamper of a friend's house to escape him.

Lewis continued to suffer from his brain fever, and with terrible arthritis added to his problems, he was having trouble at his job. Lois's maternal grandparents had moved to Sonoma, California, and in 1922 they begged the Bonseys to come down there. More jobs were available there, and Virgil and Lois were old enough to work. The family rattled through California in their Model T and arrived in Sonoma in early July, moving in with Mabelle's parents.

In the 1920s Sonoma was a small ranching and agricultural village. There were a couple of wineries in town, but the wine culture that would make Sonoma famous was a few generations in the future. After they settled in, Lois, Virgil, and their mother went out into the working world, but none of them had ever done manual labor, which was the only work available in Sonoma. Lois was now eighteen, Virgil was twenty, and Fanny and Paul, who was born in Oregon, were just fourteen and ten. So it was up to the two older children and their mother to bring in some badly needed wages.

Virgil started driving a taxi in Santa Rosa, north of town. Lois and her mother did housework around Sonoma, and Mabelle also worked in a hospital laundry. But when seasonal agricultural jobs opened up, the two women decided to give those better-paying positions a try.

Their first job was packing cherries into wooden boxes in nearby Vineburg. They had to place each cherry individually into a crate, so that when it was opened, the buyer saw only lovely, orderly red rows, like marbles. Fruit packing paid well and wasn't as strenuous as changing hotel beds or sending yellowing sheets through a laundry mangle. Lewis then heard about even better-paying jobs in Watsonville, a town on the central coast about 130 miles south of Sonoma. It was also known as Apple City for its many orchards and apple drying and packing sheds. So, in the summer of 1923, the family packed up again and spent six months as fruit tramps.

That's the phrase Lois used to describe her days among the apples; it was an archaic and quaint term for migrant workers. But she also used it as a term of affection, because although the work itself was hard, the fruit kept the family together. They lived in a cabin on a beach about seven miles southwest of Watsonville. There, Mabelle and her three oldest children worked in an apple drying facility, making about twenty-five cents per hour. They usually managed the machinery that peeled the apples, though sometimes they also sorted the raw fruit.

Lewis couldn't work at all, but he could still cook, his best and only remaining skill, and the family came home every night to a warm meal. And they were able to put by a few pennies so the kids could enjoy rides at the nearby Santa Cruz boardwalk.

When winter set in and the fruit work was over, the Bonseys returned to Sonoma. In early 1924 Lois and her mother went back to work as maids and house cleaners. In April the two women also worked as waitress and cook, respectively, for the San Francisco Seals baseball team when it came to the nearby town of Boyes Hot Springs for spring training.

Lois was now stepping out with Harvey Downey, a Sonoma electrician she'd met the previous year. On her days off, Lois jumped into Harvey's car along with a bunch of friends, and they drove an hour to one of Sonoma County's many beaches. There were always dances to go to, and she also enjoyed watching the hometown baseball team.

Lois and Harvey were married in August 1924 and moved into a little rented house next door to Harvey's parents. The following May they welcomed a son, Harvey Jr. Lois gave birth with little fuss and scandalized her mother by bouncing the baby on her stomach, singing, "Yes! We Have No Bananas," after the two of them were cleaned up.

Because she was married and a mother, Lois no longer "worked out." Harvey was now a troubleshooter for Pacific Gas & Electric Company. Although there were occasional clashes with her stern mother-in-law, Lois thrived in her new life. Or thought she did.

Lois's sister, Fanny, and brother Paul were still at home with their parents. Lois was closest to Fanny and worried about her. She had a condition that caused her to sometimes drop suddenly into a faint. In June 1927, Lois and little Harvey Jr. were visiting the family, and she saw Fanny about to have one of her spells. As she fell, Lois bent over to catch her and felt something break inside her chest. She coughed, saw blood spurting out of her mouth onto the unconscious Fanny, and fell to the floor beside her. She went straight home and called a doctor. He came to the house and gave her an opiate to put under her tongue to calm both her and the coughing. It didn't help.

Her in-laws knew what was wrong with her because they'd seen it before, though they waited for a doctor to give her the bad news. It was bad because it was tuberculosis. Lois didn't think that the cough, weight loss, and night sweats she'd been experiencing were anything to worry about. She thought these were lingering symptoms from having her tonsils removed a few weeks earlier.

Her doctor said he thought they could lick the problem. He told her to stay home in bed and gave her iron shots to build up her strength. When she was weak, he carried her from the living room onto the sunny porch to get some sunshine. He said the most important thing was to rest.

She tried, but it wasn't easy. As the summer moved into autumn, she wrapped herself in a robe and sat on the porch to watch her toddler son play in the yard and run next door to visit his grandparents. Harvey was away all day at work; in bad weather, which caused power lines to fail, he could be gone for days at a time. Lois's parents and in-laws helped take care of Harvey Jr., but leaving her child in the care of others was more upsetting than her diagnosis.

In November the doctor examined her again, but she hadn't improved. She was moving around too much, he said. She wasn't eating enough to gain the lost weight back or sleeping enough to give her lungs time to heal. The only way she could get the rest she needed was to go to a tuberculosis sanatorium. As gently as he could, he told the couple that without it, Lois would die.

They were aghast. They didn't have that kind of money. There weren't any sanatoriums near their home. They were expensive . . . the doctor stopped them in mid-panic and said there was one option. They could make an appointment with Dr. Philip King Brown in San Francisco. He had a private sanatorium in Fairfax, down in Marin County, just thirty miles away, called Arequipa. He pronounced it for them: *Air-a-KEEP-a*. It was very inexpensive because Dr. Brown had built it for poor and working women. Harvey and Lois looked at each other and the decision was made. They made an appointment for the following week.

Despite the worries over her father's chronic illness, and the hardships of her early working life, Lois was essentially a tough-minded optimist. As she readied for her appointment, she was confident that this Dr. Brown would let her into his place with the funny name that very day, so she packed a suitcase to take with her. She knew she would need a warm robe, flannel pajamas, and slippers, because even in California the winter months could be icy.

Harvey drove down the curling state highway through Marin County to the ferry terminal at Sausalito. He maneuvered the car onto the ferry and parked it, and the two of them walked to the upper deck to await the departure across San Francisco Bay. Lois, brought up on the Big Muddy, always loved water journeys. She hoped this one would have as happy an ending as the ones that filled her prairie childhood.

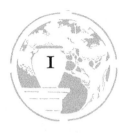

THE MAVERICK

AT 5:12 A.M., ON THE DAY of his fourth birthday, Cabot Brown woke up startled but intrigued, because his bed was rolling around the room. As his wild-eyed parents clambered over a pile of fallen bricks that partially blocked the bedroom door, he chirped, "It's just like a railroad train." His siblings were equally unruffled by what had just happened: the great San Francisco earthquake of April 18, 1906. Hillyer, age five, didn't stir until his parents grabbed him out of his crib in the corner of their bedroom. Phoebe, not yet one and sleeping in the nursery, looked at her parents and smiled when they woke her up. She then turned over and dozed off again.

After the shaking stopped and they were satisfied the children were unharmed, Dr. Philip King Brown and his wife, Helen, stood among the toppled books, bottles, and crockery and made a few quick decisions. Philip knew that a quake this size meant there would be wounded to treat, so he kissed Helen good-bye and hurried away to offer his services to local hospitals. She collected the children, their nurse, some clothes, silver, and jewelry and went to her sister's place in a safer part of the city. The Browns' home had survived the shaking, but a few days later it would succumb to dynamite, detonated to stop the fires that even now were simmering.

The flames, which raged for the next three days, took almost everything in Dr. Brown's medical office: books, instruments, X-ray machine, and laboratory. Despite the personal losses, he worked himself to collapse to help others in the following weeks. When the crisis was over and Brown could take time to recuperate, he and Helen considered their fortunes. They had to rebuild their lives, but they were wealthy and soon had a new home and office. The Browns knew how lucky they were.[1]

Dr. Philip Brown didn't need reminding that his wealth was inherited, or that it was only a generation old. Starting with little and starting over was a family tradition. His parents and grandparents had let nothing stop them from making their way up in the world, and they did it a little . . . sideways. They skirted the lines of expectations and propriety in the still unsettled West and ended up prospering beyond imagining.

Perhaps the young doctor also considered the inheritance of character in these moments. He was outwardly conventional; only those closest to him knew that a very independent thinker lurked under his suit and tie. That was also a genetic trait. Everything that Philip King Brown was, and that would become even stronger in the years after the earthquake, began with his steely, no-nonsense, and most maverick mother, Charlotte.

The funeral service at San Francisco's First Congregational Church was one of the best-attended in recent memory. It was April 21, 1904, and the unsettled, rainy weather of the previous day had turned to soft breezes and sun. There seemed to be more women than usual for a memorial event, but the woman whose body rested in the casket near the altar was more than just mother and grandmother to the small contingent of family members in the front pew. She was Dr. Charlotte Blake Brown, one of the city's first female surgeons, founder of a children's hospital and a nurses' training school, respected across the country for her skills and beloved by two generations of women who had "Dr." in front of their names because of her example. Two of Charlotte's three children also became doctors, and in their lives and practices they not only honored their mother but furthered her goal of making sure that medicine did not treat women as an afterthought.

We don't know if Charlotte Brown's early life was woven into the eulogy given that day, but it should have been. She had the kind of childhood any boy would envy, and it perfectly explains her barrier-shattering career choice. Sandwiched between two brothers, Charles Jr. and Thomas, she was born in Philadelphia on December 21, 1846. Her parents, Charles Blake and Charlotte Farrington, were natives of Maine and were both trained as teachers, but Charles was also a licensed minister and took a few classes at a Philadelphia medical college. He was the oldest son of his father's first marriage, and it is no surprise that he received a first-class education. First sons often got the lion's share of any available opportunities, but they also tended to shoulder more family responsibilities because of it. Charles, however, did not. He had feet that itched to travel and a mind that was always eager for new experiences.

He went alone to California in 1849, crossing Mexico first to do some preaching, and then tried his hand at gold mining, which, as the cliché goes, did not pan out. After being away from home for two years, he returned to Philadelphia in the fall of 1851 to fetch his wife and three children back to California, which he still thought had something to offer. They traveled across the Isthmus of Panama, the shortest route that easterners could take to get to the Golden State. The trip involved a steamship voyage from New York to the Caribbean side of the isthmus, followed by a boat ride up the Chagres River. Charlotte often told her children about being carried on the shoulders of native Panamanians as they navigated the waters. The final leg of the trip was an eighteen-mile mule ride to Panama City, on the Pacific. There, the family boarded a steamer, which deposited them on the San Francisco docks in October.[2]

Charles and wife Charlotte opened a boys' school in the town of Benicia, across the bay from San Francisco. They had another girl, Mary Ellen, in November 1853. But the promise of fulfillment in the golden land went very sour in 1854. In February, five-year-old Thomas died of croup, and little Mary Ellen died in August.

Whether escaping unbearable grief or from a desire to practice his original profession, Charles gathered up the family again and took them to Chile, where he got a job ministering to a congregation of Americans and Europeans, many of them miners from Cornwall. According to family lore, their ship was blown off course and they spent a short time in Tahiti while they waited for repairs. The Blakes stayed in Chile until 1857. Charles then decided to go back to Pennsylvania, where ministerial fields and educational opportunities for the children were richer. The Blakes welcomed another daughter in August 1859, but like her tiny sister, she did not survive long, passing away in November 1860, leaving Charlotte and Charles Jr. as the only Blake children.

When the Civil War broke out, Charles Sr. enlisted in the army and was assigned as chaplain to Maj. Gen. John C. Frémont, the 1856 antislavery presidential candidate, now in command of troops in Missouri. Charles then saw action commanding African American troops in South Carolina and Florida, where he received a head wound in the Battle of Olustee in February 1864. He later served as a hospital chaplain in Chattanooga. War or no war, educating their children was still a priority for Charles and his wife. After leaving Phillips Exeter Academy in New Hampshire in 1861, Charles, Jr. enrolled at Yale. In the fall of 1862, Charlotte, schooled nearer home in Pennsylvania, went to upstate New York and entered Elmira College. She was not quite sixteen years old.[3]

The fact that their daughter attended college at all speaks to the value that Charles and Charlotte Blake put not only on education but on education for women. There were other universities for women in the mid-Atlantic region, such as Mount Holyoke and Vassar. But Elmira was the first college founded specifically to grant undergraduate degrees to women, which it did from the first day it opened its doors in 1855. Less than a decade later it was hailed for its educational rigor. Elmira attracted women such as Charlotte's classmate Olivia Langdon, daughter of one of the founding members. She later married Mark Twain.

Charles Jr. graduated in the spring of 1865, and Charlotte received her bachelor's degree in 1866. Before returning home she posed for a commemorative class photograph. At first glance it is the typical portrait of a modest twenty-year-old woman of the mid-nineteenth century. Her dark hair is brushed back from a center part, curled into a large chignon that peeks around the back of her head. A stiff white collar fastened with a circular brooch sits atop a simple dress with buttons down the front. Charlotte's eyes are dark and deep set, and an earring seems to dangle from one earlobe.

But then you notice the smile.

It's not the shy spasm of a woman unsure of herself or one who is uncomfortable in front of a camera, wondering what she is supposed to do while the exposure is made. It's a confident and almost amused smile, as though she is thinking of something interesting but hasn't decided to share it. Thanks to the years of travel with her fidgety father, and exposure to cultures outside the United States, Charlotte was already more sophisticated than many of her friends. It's easy to imagine the stories she told about the ocean voyages she took before she was eleven years old and the colorful people she encountered in California and South America. But all Elmira women were strong and independent, and four years spent among them shaped Charlotte's character even more at a very crucial time.

Charles Blake was still a military chaplain, and when he got new orders in May 1866, the family moved to Arizona Territory (minus Charles Jr., who joined them later). The army posted Blake as chaplain at Fort Whipple, just outside Prescott, the territorial capital. The Blakes took the Panama route again, a much easier trip than it had been in 1851. They stepped off the New York steamer right onto the Panama Railroad and rode in comfort the entire fifty miles to Panama City. There, they boarded the steamship *Colorado* and arrived in San Francisco on September 12. Another boat took them to the southern California port of Wilmington, and from there they went overland on the Mojave Road—with a military escort.

Traveling the Mojave Road was dangerous, thanks to recent agitations between the military, miners, and the territory's indigenous people, who were generally called Apaches no matter what tribe they came from. A rickety wagon took the family across the desert, where they stayed in rude adobe accommodations at army posts sprinkled along the way: Camp Cady (near Barstow, California), Marl Springs (now in the Mojave National Preserve), and Hardyville (Bullhead City, Arizona).[4]

Whipple was a fairly new fort in the very new town of Prescott, created in 1864 as the capital of recently created Arizona Territory. It's unclear whether the Blakes lived at the fort or in town, but Charles had congregations in both places. Charles Jr. took up farming, and by July 1867 he had thirty-seven acres of corn planted in the nearby Whipple Valley.

Charlotte kept busy too. On February 18, 1867, she opened a school for the roughly twenty-five children who lived in and around town. The cost was two dollars per week, payable in advance. It's hard to know if this was her real vocation, if her father talked her into it, or if she just needed something to do.[5] But a few months later, Charlotte gave up her school when she took on another project: marriage.

Like the Blakes, Henry Adams Brown was from Maine, born on April 3, 1842, the fifth son to survive to adulthood. Henry's brother William was twelve years older and was a westerner by 1860, serving as the county treasurer in the Sierra Nevada town of Oroville, California. In 1864 he moved down to Napa, where he took a job as city postmaster. Henry also decided to move West, but he ended up in Arizona. How and when he got there is unknown, but we can pick up his trail in the spring of 1866.

By this time he was in business with a man named William T. Silverthorn. Brown & Silverthorn was a wholesale hardware and dry goods firm, and its inventory included fabrics, clothing, ribbons, boots, and other soft goods, in addition to shovels and nails. The men spent much of their time in and around Prescott and could have met the Blake family either in town or out at Fort Whipple, where they may have had government contracts.[6]

However whirlwind their romance may (or may not) have been, Henry Brown and Charlotte Blake were married at Whipple on September 12, 1867. Charles performed the ceremony, which was one of his final tasks at the fort. He had been ordered to report to Camp McDowell, about 120 miles away, northeast of Phoenix. The fort needed a chaplain, and he and his wife took up residence there in October.[7]

The newly married Browns stayed behind in Prescott, and by October Charlotte was pregnant with their first child. At some point they made the decision to leave the territory and move to Napa, to be near Henry's brother and his wife. Despite the presence of children running around Prescott, they thought Arizona was no place to start a family. When they headed west, Henry and Charlotte were grateful that they were accompanied out of the area by local troops until it was safe enough for them to go on alone. Years later Charlotte told her children that one of the soldiers gave her a warning as they got under way: "If we are attacked by Indians, the first bullet will be for you."

Henry and Charlotte arrived safely in Napa well before July 19, 1868, the day their daughter Adelaide was born. Charlotte had help on hand to bring her first child into the world: her sister-in-law and, if she needed him, a well-known local doctor named Charles Nichell.

When Henry and Charlotte moved to Napa it was a thriving mercantile hub with mills, retail stores, saloons, tanneries, newspapers, schools, and a library, all fed by transportation via the Napa River and the Napa Valley Railroad. Henry took a job as a store clerk. Charlotte settled into life as a wife and mother, and got to know her new in-laws. By the end of March 1869, Charlotte's parents were also living in town, and her brother would soon join them. Charles had left the army, and the couple wanted to be near their granddaughter and an imminent new arrival, as Charlotte was pregnant with her second child. The Browns welcomed a son, named Philip King, on June 24, 1869. Another girl, Harriet, arrived on January 12, 1871, and sometime that year Henry got a new job as a bookkeeper for a local government tax collector.[8]

Motherhood wasn't the only thing on Charlotte's mind. The Blake family's activities and ambitions went in two directions—education and medicine—occasionally at the same time. Charles managed to not only study both of these fields but had also added the ministry to his list. Charlotte's mother was a trained teacher and helped run a boys' school in California. Charles Jr. was planning to go to medical school in nearby San Francisco. Well-educated Charlotte had tried teaching, but by the time Philip was born, she had made up her strong Blake mind and set her sights on a profession. This was rare for a woman in 1870s America, and the path she chose was even more unusual: Charlotte was going to be a doctor.

~

Women were doctors before there were medical schools.

For centuries, mothers, wives, aunts, and grandmothers were responsible for the health of their families and communities. They grew herbs, delivered one another's babies, made poultices, brewed tonics, and bandaged wounds. But formal education in medicine, once it came along, was reserved for men only. In nineteenth-century America, bleeding with leeches and instruments and purging with emetics were the two goalposts of knowledge, even in medical schools. A man could hang up his shingle after simply following another doctor around and attending a series of lectures. After the Civil War some men tried to elevate medicine to a higher level and move beyond such "heroic" measures, but there wasn't anything to replace them with. Schools didn't have clinical facilities, and the germ theory of medicine was decades in the future.

New therapies emerged, but they competed with traditional medicine rather than improving on it. Hydrotherapy, homeopathy, hypnotism, herbalism, and phrenology (studying the shape of the skull) had many followers, and some practitioners opened their own schools. These institutions welcomed women into the classroom, which traditional medical schools did not.

The first woman to struggle through the prejudice against female physicians and get a medical degree was Elizabeth Blackwell, who graduated from New York's Geneva Medical College in 1849. After spending time studying in Europe, she came back to New York and opened her own practice in 1853. She founded a dispensary, or clinic, designed especially to treat the poor and where she could see patients on her own terms. In 1857 she opened the New York Infirmary for Women and Children, which gave training, experience, and sisterhood to female doctors when they graduated from the medical schools that were now grudgingly admitting them.

Another generation would have to pass before an African American woman held a medical degree. This milestone belongs to Rebecca Lee Crumpler, who graduated from the New England Female Medical College in 1864. After the Civil War she gave her skills to the Freedmen's Bureau in Richmond, Virginia, treating the many ills of former slaves trying to find their way in the postwar world. She also wrote an acclaimed medical text titled *A Book of Medical Discourses in Two Parts* in 1883.[9]

Women who battered through the doors of medicine were doing so as part of a larger movement of social revolution and self-determination. Dress reform (getting rid of layers of restrictive and unhealthy clothing), suffrage, and an attention to the health of the poor were the flip side of what was considered a woman's natural role.

But going to school and becoming a doctor was just too much. Some men said that practicing medicine with other "professionals" would put women in competition with men, subject them to the immorality of the outside world, unfeminize them, and, by default, feminize men and the medical profession itself. Modesty would be outraged if women cut bodies open, were exposed to the indelicacy of bodily functions, or saw unclothed men who were not their husbands. Not only that, educating women was a waste of time, some said. Why spend time and money on someone who would eventually get married, have children, and not even use her degree?[10]

Women had answers for these arguments. They reminded their critics that women had always been the doctors in the family and had seen plenty of blood, flesh, and bodily functions. They added that if marriage and childbearing were their lot in life, being more educated about medicine would make them better wives and mothers. It took a long time for the message to trickle down into actual education though. And this was especially true in California, making Charlotte's decision harder to put into action.

The state's first medical school was founded in 1858 by Dr. Elias Samuel Cooper. Called the Medical Department of the University of the Pacific, it was chartered by that university, located near Santa Clara, south of San Francisco. Lectures, dissection, and courses in toxicology, gynecology, and surgery filled the curriculum. When Cooper died in 1862, the college fell into disarray, and the board of trustees eventually suspended its courses. But a new institution, the Toland Medical School, opened in the fall of 1864 in San Francisco's North Beach district. It was run by and named for Dr. Hubert H. Toland, a South Carolina native who had come to the state during the gold rush.

Toland was pleased with its quick success, but he had higher aspirations. The University of California had founded its Berkeley campus in 1868, and president Daniel Coit Gilman, who was a strong supporter of the sciences, worked with Toland to merge both colleges into a medical school headquartered in San Francisco. Although Toland threw a fit because the new school wouldn't be named for him and then threatened to build a rival college, he relented after the university endowed a chair in his name. The new Medical Department of the University of California opened in 1873, and one of its early students was Charlotte's brother, Charles Jr.[11]

The University of the Pacific and Toland had not admitted women, but the University of California did. So when Toland became part of the UC system, women were allowed to apply for medical degrees. The first two women who tried to get into the school were rejected, but when the regents heard about this they forced the issue, and Lucy Wanzer enrolled as the first woman in the medical school in 1876.[12]

This didn't help Charlotte though. The desire to train as a doctor began brewing in her mind soon after Philip's birth in 1869 and was a fully formed plan by the time Harriet was born two years later. California's medical schools were not ready for her. But she had an ally in Napa, and thanks to one of the ways that medicine was studied in the United States, she was able to get started while she was still at home. And that was because she had Dr. Charles Nichell.

Born in Germany, Nichell emigrated to the United States when he was a young man and later earned his medical degree in New York. He then married and moved to Napa with his wife in the late 1860s. Sometime after Charlotte gave birth to her son Philip, Nichell took Charlotte on as his apprentice, becoming her mentor or, to use the proper term, preceptor.

Medical apprenticeship sounds strange to us today. Treating medicine as a learned craft under a master, like shoemaking, doesn't seem like the best way to train good doctors. But in the nineteenth century a preceptor taking a student under his wing was not only traditional, it was a method that medical schools valued highly. Especially for women. Prospective female students had a better chance of getting into a college with some training behind them and a letter from a preceptor in their hands.

This relationship had no set pattern, and it was up to the preceptor to decide the best way to help his student. Reading his medical books was almost always part of the plan, even if the apprentice accompanied the doctor on rounds or observed surgery later on. In Charlotte's case her personal life probably dictated what her work with Dr. Nichell looked like. Family members said that she read anatomy with him, and with three children under the age of five to care for, reading is probably all that she did for a while. Given her intelligence and commitment, that was enough.[13]

She had a very specific place in mind when she was ready to start her formal studies in 1872. There were a few women-friendly universities to choose from, but the first, and the best, was the one she settled on: the Woman's Medical College of Pennsylvania, in her hometown of Philadelphia.

In 1850 a group of liberal Quaker physicians and businessmen decided to open a school where women could learn medicine. Many of these men had already been preceptors for Quaker women, a few of whom were the daughters of the college's founders. They saw a void and decided to fill it, calling their new institution the Female Medical College of Pennsylvania.

They made sure the faculty was composed of medically orthodox practitioners—no hydrotherapists or homeopathists for them. Some graduates later became professors themselves. A few of the college's male instructors were ridiculed by their peers and dropped away, so the early years were marked by struggles to find teachers. Prejudice also showed itself in other ways. Medical journals would not publish the college's ads, and local hospitals refused to let women do clinical studies in their wards. But the Quaker founders were used to opposition and kept the doors open.

In 1861 Ann Preston, who was in the first graduating class, established the Woman's Hospital so that students could get the clinical experience they needed, and by 1869 Philadelphia's hospitals had relented and finally let women use their facilities. In 1866 Preston became the college's dean, and in 1867 she changed the name to the Woman's Medical College of Pennsylvania.

Preston had a unique definition of what a medical education should be. She believed in a broad, liberal grounding, and she took students to lectures given by cultural celebrities such as suffragist Lucy Stone and transcendentalist Ralph Waldo Emerson. The female faculty were much-needed role models, and in contrast to the situation at coeducational medical schools, academic life at the college was as supportive as it was rigorous. One graduate later wrote that a woman's medical education was not complete unless she spent at least one term at the Woman's Medical College.[14]

Even after the college and its students were accepted by most patients and peers, some doctors still thought the idea of a female physician unacceptable, even scandalous. One man who attended its graduation ceremony in 1876 lumped the new doctors together with other women reformers, calling them "ill-favored, near-sighted, vinegar-tempered, odd-costumed, eccentric and unfeminine."[15]

Only a self-aware, supremely confident young woman would take this path, which Charlotte certainly was, thanks to her parents' deep belief in the importance of education for women. They championed her decision to go to medical school, of course. They didn't spend all that time and money educating their daughter just to suddenly turn conventional.

How Charlotte paid for her education, and the travel expenses that went along with it, is a mystery. The Blakes were able to send both of their children to excellent colleges a decade earlier, even though Charles was just an army chaplain. Not only that, he had resigned from the army by the time he and his wife moved to Napa. Henry Brown's bookkeeping job wasn't lucrative either, so how did Charlotte do it? Her parents probably had family funds from relatives back in Maine to tap into, but it's impossible to know. Charlotte could have attended the University of California's medical school in San Francisco along with her brother if she didn't have enough money to head east to Philadelphia. But she would have had to wait four long years for the university to admit women, and she was lucky to have the financing to match her ambition.

Once she decided to go to Philadelphia for training, Charlotte's plans began to come together. Part of that planning involved her children, and this was the hardest part of the entire endeavor. To get her degree, Charlotte would need to be away from home for two years. Travel between Philadelphia and California was much easier by this time thanks to the transcontinental railroad, so she could come home between terms, though we don't know if she did. But even contemplating the months she would be away from the children must have given her pause. Her husband and parents would have to take charge of every aspect of their lives: education, nurturing, birthday celebrations, illnesses. But she had to set emotion aside to meet a larger goal. She knew this would be a good example for her children later in life.

Charlotte's daughter Adelaide wrote an article about her mother in 1925 and had this to say about her time away from the family. "For their faith in her ambitions enough can not be said for the co-operation of her husband and parents."[16] Charlotte's maternal grandmother, however, was a different story. When she heard about the plan, she wrote Charlotte's mother an agitated letter from Maine. How, she asked, was she supposed to tell her friends that Lottie was studying medicine?

Like most of her fellow students, Charlotte already had a college degree, so once she arrived on campus in the spring of 1872, the setting and expectations were not new. The subject matter was, but thanks to Dr. Nichell, Charlotte was very well prepared. The companionship and support of her years at Elmira were re-created in Philadelphia, and she thrived as she worked hard at her studies.

∾

Charlotte went off to medical school believing that she had left her family in good hands. Her parents stepped in to help with the children so that Charlotte could get her education, and her father, Charles, may have brought in some extra money by teaching school. But husband Henry was another story.

No diary or letters survive to tell us how Henry felt about his wife disappearing for two years, leaving him to share a home with his in-laws and three young children. Henry Brown's character had already revealed itself when he left Arizona without paying property taxes owed to Yavapai County and refused to pay other debts until forced to by the courts. Even so, what happened on the afternoon of June 21, 1873, seems very shocking.

At noon that day, Henry left his office to go home for lunch. As he walked down Coombs Street near Clay, deep in today's downtown Napa, a local tinsmith named Ned Kimball began to follow him, holding a double-barreled shotgun in one hand. A crowd of locals and a writer for the *Napa Reporter* trailed behind, figuring that something interesting was about to happen. As Henry crossed the street, Kimball stopped, raised up the shotgun, aimed, and fired.

A volley of quail shot hit Henry in the back, splattering across his coat. He hollered, reeled completely around, and then ran toward his home a block away. Before Henry could get in the door, Kimball let loose the other barrel, but missed him. Brown staggered into his house, and Kimball put the gun over his shoulder and then walked calmly to the courthouse to turn himself in.

Henry was covered with tiny lead shot from the back of his neck to his calves, and the valise he carried was perforated and covered with blood. Quail shot is so small that although he was in a lot of pain, his life was never in danger. Charles called for Dr. Nichell, who came over to remove the shot and treat the open wounds.

The newspaper reporter had followed Henry from the scene of the shooting and actually managed to get into the house. He gave his paper a firsthand account of what he saw: "Henry Brown got to his house, where we found him walking about the room. His back was bespattered with quail-shot, one of which we picked out of his linen coat, and his left hand was wrapped in a bloody handkerchief. Asking him if he was badly hurt, he replied: 'I expect he has killed me.' Looking at the tiny speck of flattened lead we held between our forefinger and thumb, we failed to concur."[17]

Kimball's reason for shooting Henry was distasteful and embarrassing: he claimed that Henry had been sleeping with his wife. In fact, Kimball had already warned Henry to stay away from her. By the end of June Kimball was living in a hotel instead of his home, and after weeks of brooding on the situation, gunfire seemed the only solution. Although the local newspapers said the affair was just a rumor, the subtext condemned Henry as a homewrecker. And Kimball was apparently never charged or brought to trial for the shooting.

Henry recovered, but of course someone had to write to Charlotte to tell her what had happened. She was still in the East, and however adversely this event may have affected her heart, her studies did not suffer. What Henry or his father-in-law told the children, however, will never be known.

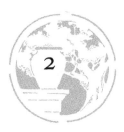

THE DRS. BROWN

CHARLOTTE RECEIVED HER MD at the Woman's Medical College graduation ceremony on March 13, 1874, along with the other seventeen women in her class. She then said her good-byes and made a speedy return to Napa. Adelaide, Philip, and Harriet were now six, five, and three years old, young enough to have adapted to Charlotte's absence and then to readapt to her return.

Henry and Charlotte had to remake their marriage too. There is no record of what he said to explain the shooting, or whether Charlotte believed it. But one fact is indisputable: despite her previous fertility and her still-young age, she never had another child.

Husband and children had a couple of months to fold her back into their lives, and then the entire family, including Charlotte's parents, packed up and moved to the one place where an ambitious, dedicated female doctor could have a career and kick aside the barriers for her sisters: San Francisco.

Early visitors to San Francisco reveled in its beautiful bay setting, cleansing winds, and moderate temperatures (though the foggy summers were a bit of a surprise). But natural beauty did not translate into robust health for residents, especially after the gold rush drew thousands of people to the city's shores and crammed them into hastily erected homes and commercial buildings. Cholera and other gastrointestinal illnesses stalked residents, and despair over dashed hopes caused many suicides. Fires in the 1850s led to better-built structures, and the Civil War brought greater prosperity, but it was the years after the war that helped city leaders make better medical decisions.

In the late 1860s and early 1870s, San Francisco existed in a strange middle ground between its gold rush childhood and the coming maturity of the Gilded

Age. The city was now in early adulthood, mostly settled and looking toward the future but still immature enough to be lured by the thrill of risk-taking behavior. San Franciscans wanted personal and commercial success, and they wanted to have a good time getting it. Two events brought both the potential and the reality of this kind of success, but not everyone got to share in the benefits.

The completion of the transcontinental railroad in 1869 brought an end to Pacific coast isolation. Steamers still puffed into the bay from Panama, bringing dry goods, hardware, miners, capitalists, and scalawags, but the railroad gave the city's merchants and wealthier citizens another way to get around. It also increased San Francisco's importance as a distribution center for consumer goods.

However, the men who had built the railroad now needed new jobs, and they flocked into town to look for them. It was a terrible time for labor, made worse because newly unemployed Chinese men also needed work, and they began to fill up already crowded Chinatown. Racism and inflammatory rhetoric about labor being taken away from white men made a difficult situation intolerable and even murderous. Outside the city, thousands of acres of land that could have been used for farms or ranches were now owned by the railroad, making agricultural work also harder to find.

The rush to Nevada after multiple silver strikes created a frenzy for stock buying and speculation in the mid-1860s. Mark Twain happened to be in San Francisco at the time, and he wrote about this fervid atmosphere in *Roughing It*: "Stocks went rising; speculation went mad; bankers, merchants, lawyers, doctors, mechanics, laborers, even the very washer-women and servant girls, were putting up their earnings on silver stocks, and every sun that rose in the morning went down on paupers enriched and rich men beggared. What a gambling carnival it was."[1]

This edifice eventually crashed, and more destitute people began to flow through the city's streets, which were unspeakably filthy. Unemployment breeds poverty, which in its turn breeds illness. In 1874, the year the Browns moved to San Francisco, 4,044 people died within the city limits. Most of these deaths were due to what were then called zymotic, or infectious, diseases: typhus, typhoid, smallpox, scarlet fever, measles, cholera, and diphtheria.[2]

The city provided a lot of business for its doctors, but only a few of them were women. When Charlotte and her family moved to San Francisco in late April 1874, twenty women were listed as physicians in the city directory. They had their own category—"Physicians-Female"—instead of being mixed in with the regular "Physicians" column. Among them were one spiritual healer, three women who were practicing "hygienic" medicine, four who specialized in the "water cure," and nineteen homeopaths. Also on hand were thirty midwives and eighty-three nurses, most of whom can be identified by their names as women or who were listed with only their initials.

And the category called simply "Physicians" listed more than five hundred male doctors.

Dr. Charlotte Brown's overarching goal was to live a life of service, using medicine as her vehicle. But Charlotte didn't want to be just another "female" name in the city directory, and this meant dealing with the legions of male physicians in town. She didn't mind that these men expected her to focus her practice on women and children. On the contrary: she wanted to make the health of women and children a priority. She didn't know it, but the stake she placed in the ground would affect the health of the city's women well beyond her death.

The Brown family settled into a home just a block away from a former garbage dump that was now a park called Union Square. A little farther west, where the poor tended to congregate, the houses were a bit shabbier. This area would soon be called the Tenderloin. Her patients were therefore drawn from the middle class as well as the most poverty-stricken, which was a selling point for the location. There, she saw everything from simple sprains to difficult childbirths. The area was also affordable. Henry got a job working for the banking division of Wells, Fargo & Co., which had a popular and thriving express business linked up with railroads all over the country.[3]

Charlotte—known by convention as Mrs. Dr. Brown—got to know many of her fellow female physicians, and within a few months of starting her practice, she realized that mothers and babies could not get adequate care in the city's hospitals. She started to talk about this problem with her colleagues, and in March 1875, Charlotte, Dr. Martha Bucknell, and ten society women (who provided the funding) opened the Pacific Dispensary for Women and Children. The dispensary gave free care to patients, charging a small fee only for medicines. Five years later, Dr. Brown opened a training school for nurses as part of the dispensary's mission, the first its kind west of the Rockies. She also found time in her schedule to give free medical care and advice to many San Francisco charities, such as the Young Women's Christian Association.[4]

The commitment she made when she first moved to San Francisco saw its fruition in the many ways she helped mothers, young women, and children with medical care and with education. Newly minted doctors interned at her hospital, came to Charlotte for advice, attended her surgeries, and found in her the kind of mentor they needed. It was easier to be a woman doctor than it had been in the past, but resentments still lingered.

She influenced another group of young people too, and they were the most important of all. Despite her busy professional and charitable schedule, Charlotte brought up her children to understand that their education and the advantages they were given obliged them to always think about the welfare of others. They did not disappoint her.

Charlotte and Henry Brown were able to give Adelaide, Philip, and Harriet something that their mother had not experienced: an uneventful childhood. Charlotte had grown up with adventures few young people could match. Living in places such as Chile and Arizona Territory gave her a curiosity that followed her into maturity. She never tired of learning, especially new medical techniques. Henry didn't leave Maine until he was a young adult, but his leaving at all meant that life on the Eastern Seaboard was not for him. The Browns, now comfortable and prospering, softened the edges of their children's lives, determined that the difficulties of their own youths would not have to be repeated.

However, this did not mean that the little Browns were timid. They were brought up on tales of crossing rivers, oceans, and deserts; of conflicts with Indians and the sound of a bugle calling soldiers to reveille. These stories quietly schooled them in the values of being adaptable to new situations and of pride in being pioneers in new places.

For the girls especially, Charlotte's departure for medical school and her deep commitment to her career allowed them to see that they also had choices, despite their gender. They saw their mother at her work every day, and sometimes saw her called away from the dinner table to help a woman in labor or tend to another woman's sick child. Adelaide and Harriet saw their mother's joy in her profession, and just having a mother with a profession was a lesson in itself. There were lessons for Philip too. Women belonged in medicine, and their female patients deserved the best medical care they could get.

All the Brown children were educated in San Francisco's public grammar schools. After graduation, Adelaide and Harriet enrolled at Smith College in Northampton, Massachusetts. Considering that their mother had been educated at two women's colleges, it makes sense that she would steer her daughters in that direction, even though the University of California admitted women with little prejudice by this time. Adelaide graduated with a bachelor of arts in 1888, and Harriet with a literature degree in 1891. Both women returned to San Francisco and then went in different directions.

Adelaide had also decided on a medical career, but she wanted to take a vacation before moving on, and in the summer after her graduation from Smith, she and a friend went to Yosemite National Park. They could have afforded a stay at the luxurious Ahwahnee Hotel but decided to rough it by taking a tent cabin at what was then called Camp Curry, near Glacier Point. One night a bear wandered into the tent, and when Adelaide's friend, Amanda, started screaming, Adelaide jumped up, grabbed a broom, and brandished it at the bear, which turned tail and ran. One of Adelaide's nephews later wrote about this family legend, and in his mind his formidable aunt, still wearing her nightgown and waving the broom, chased the bear across Yosemite Valley in the manner of the Headless Horseman pursuing Ichabod Crane.[5]

After her summer adventure, Adelaide Brown enrolled at Cooper Medical School, which was the revived version of the school founded by Dr. Elias Samuel Cooper in 1858. By 1872 the Medical Department of the University of the Pacific had been reorganized as the Medical College of the Pacific and was affiliated with San Francisco's City College. In 1882 Dr. Levi Cooper Lane, who was Cooper's nephew, donated a building to the school, and its name was changed again to honor the memory of his uncle.

Adelaide graduated from Cooper in 1892 and then interned at Northeastern Hospital in Boston, later going to Vienna to study at European gynecological clinics. In 1894 she came back to San Francisco, moved into her parents' home, and joined her mother's medical practice, specializing in the treatment of women and children. There were now two female Drs. Brown in San Francisco.[6]

Meanwhile, Philip King Brown also decided to go into the family business, and like his sisters, he went east for his education. He aimed just as high as they did. He chose Harvard.

He enrolled there in 1886 and received his undergraduate degree in 1890. He returned home to San Francisco for the summer and then turned right around and went back to enter medical school. Even though he already had one Harvard degree on his wall, he needed to pass exams in a daunting collection of subjects to get accepted as a med student: English, Latin, physics, chemistry, and one elective, either French, German, algebra, plane geometry, or botany. Once enrolled, he attended lectures and clinical demonstrations, and although the normal course of study took four years, Philip graduated in three.

He came back again to San Francisco and got his California medical license in June 1893. His grandfather had died earlier that year, and his grandmother had passed in 1887, so Charlotte was now the family matriarch. In early 1894 she also had to plan the funeral of her brother, who had died suddenly while tending a patient. But later that year the Browns were able to celebrate when Harriet married Boston attorney Herbert Darling. She moved east with her husband and took up woman suffrage instead of medicine.

Philip King Brown now had his own practice in a small building with offices and furnished rooms near Union Square, though he still lived in the family home. This made sense; like his sister Adelaide, he was unmarried, under thirty, and still new to his profession.

He began his career by volunteering to be the visiting physician for the Associated Charities. Founded in 1889, it was San Francisco's first general public relief organization with no ties to any specific religion. This wasn't Philip Brown's only foray into the world of philanthropy and big causes, however. One of the first organizations he'd been involved with, even before he hung out his shingle, was the San Francisco Boys' Club. Its mission was similar to its mission today: provide a safe place for boys to meet, play, and learn. He was one of the club's founders when it was getting off the ground in 1891, and in 1893 and 1894 he was secretary of its board of managers.[7] While serving on the board and hanging out with the kids, he met many interesting and influential people, and one of them was destined to change his life.

She was Phoebe Apperson Hearst.

~

Anyone who has lived in the San Francisco Bay Area or studied at the University of California at Berkeley knows Phoebe Hearst's name. She was one of the greatest philanthropists of the nineteenth century, and in contrast to her money-spending peers—Carnegie and Rockefeller, for example—she gave away her money almost exclusively in California and the West.

Born in Franklin County, Missouri, in 1842, she was raised by Randolph and Drusilla Apperson, poor but thoughtful parents who taught her housework, horsemanship, and the tenets of the Presbyterian Church. She went to a Presbyterian academy and earned a teaching certificate so that she could bring money into the family home and, even more importantly, gain some financial independence. Then, in 1860, George Hearst walked into her life.

Actually, he had already been there. The Hearsts were the Appersons' neighbors, and George Hearst, born in 1820, left Missouri for California in 1850, hoping to make a life for himself that did not involve farming. Mining intrigued him, but he had very little luck and at times turned to store-keeping.

Strangely enough even to him, his heart was deep down in the earth. When he was nearly broke in 1859, he heard about some new ore strikes in Nevada, where men were finding an abundance of gold as well as a strange bluish ore. He invested in a few of the mines there and was astonished when he found out that the odd-colored rock was silver. The Washoe silver rush was soon on, and Hearst was riding its topmost wave.

He returned to Missouri when he heard his mother was ill and reacquainted himself with the nearby families. Little Phoebe Apperson, who had been eight years old when he went away, was now eighteen and a dark-eyed beauty. Hearst had been thinking of getting married, and Phoebe not only suited him, she was more than happy to leave Missouri for the adventurous life this newly rich man could give her. They were married on June 15, 1862, and five months later were settled in San Francisco. The Hearsts moved into a hotel/apartment complex and on April 29, 1863, their son and only child, William Randolph Hearst, was born.

Phoebe Hearst threw herself into a life of culture and refinement, filling her library with books on history and art. She was a familiar face at the city's many cultural events and was soon a patron of artists and literary figures. Before the 1880s, she often donated money to deserving individuals, but after her return from a trip to Europe she widened her scope and moved from individual charity to systematic philanthropy, using her money to change society as well as lives. She began to fund orphanages and convalescent homes and was especially interested in the new kindergarten movement.

The Hearsts moved to Washington, D.C., in 1886 when George was appointed to fill the term of deceased California senator John Miller. He was elected in his own right the following year. Phoebe Hearst re-created her San Francisco home and influence while living on the opposite coast. She believed that education had many faces and that it was especially important for women to be exposed to culture and learning even if they didn't have the opportunity to go to college. She began to mentor the young people who came within her orbit, whether through friends or the institutions she championed.

George Hearst died in Washington on February 28, 1891, and at his wife's request, his body was sent back to San Francisco for the funeral. After it was over, Phoebe left the city to recover and to begin the next phase of her life as the West's most generous philanthropist. George had left her his entire fortune, which would be a thorn in the side of her brilliant but unruly son in the coming years. But Will Hearst's loss was California's gain. Phoebe continued to mentor girls and young women, and she gave her time and money to many causes in San Francisco. One of them was the Boys' Club.[8]

Phoebe Hearst and Philip King Brown met sometime after he began serving on the Boys' Club board in 1893. His mother probably introduced the two of them, as Dr. Charlotte Brown's hospital for children was one of Phoebe's charities. Over the next two years they spent a lot of time together, thanks to their mutual interests in organizations that served the poor.

∽

Philip King Brown knew that if he wanted to advance in his career he would need to follow his sister's example and do postgraduate study in Europe. Doctors who could afford it spent months or years in Germany or Vienna, where long-established medical schools educated students in the most up-to-date methods and philosophies. From March 1895 to February 1896 Philip studied in Berlin and Göttingen. In April he returned home, where he jumped into both his career and his social life, hitting a stride that must have impressed his overachieving mother. A few months after returning to the city and moving into the family home, Philip King Brown rented rooms for his medical practice once again.

Despite the hours needed to get into the swing of his new career, Brown managed to enjoy his leisure time, which he spent with some of San Francisco's most well-known and occasionally notorious people. One of them was his Boys' Club cofounder, Gelett Burgess.

Born in Boston in 1866, Burgess was an artist but took a degree in engineering. He moved west and taught topographical drawing at the University of California–Berkeley.[9] That career came to an end in 1894 with an incident that presaged his future career as a humorist. During the early hours of January 2, Burgess and a few friends waded into a water fountain at the corner of Market and California Streets in San Francisco. The fountain featured a statue of temperance advocate Dr. Henry Cogswell. Using ropes that they then left at the scene, the young men pulled the statue down and took off before the policeman on the beat saw them. (Whether the statue was toppled because of Cogswell's anti-alcohol stance or because it was just ugly is still being debated.)[10] Although newspapers reported that no one knew who the vandals were, Burgess's employers at the university somehow found out and he was out of a job.

His teaching career over, Burgess turned to satire in print and in 1895 founded a magazine called the *Lark*, along with Bruce Porter, another Massachusetts native who had made his way to California. A year older than Burgess,

Porter was a stained-glass artist, landscape designer, and critic, with the same bohemian streak as his magazine coconspirator. The *Lark* sent very unserious poetry out into the world, and even its appearance was unusual: Burgess and Porter printed their work on pages of yellowish bamboo fiber.[11] It was in these pages that Burgess published one of the silliest poems ever written.

> I never saw a Purple Cow,
> I never hope to see one,
> But I can tell you, anyhow,
> I'd rather see than be one!

The *New York Times* reviewed the first issue when it came out in May 1895, dubbing *The Lark*'s founders "*les jeunes*, those of California, forsooth, and delightfully young they are."[12]

Burgess and Porter were not alone in their goofy sensibilities. They were part of a larger circle of accomplished men who thrived in turn-of-the-century San Francisco. In essence, they were the city's first counterculture. The group included painter Ernest Peixotto, architect Willis Polk, calligrapher and author Porter Garnett, poet Yone Noguchi, and writer Frank Norris, author of the book *McTeague: A Story of San Francisco*, which Erich von Stroheim made into the film *Greed* in 1924. These men adopted the moniker bestowed on them by the *New York Times* and soon referred to themselves as Les Jeunes (The Youth).[13]

Philip knew Burgess well, though we don't know how they met and ended up founding the Boys' Club together. Despite his reputation for pranking and oddball poetry, Burgess was seriously committed to the club and served for years as its president. Through Burgess, Philip met many of the eclectic members of Les Jeunes. On May 1, 1896, he attended a dinner they held at Martinelli's, a saloon in the Commercial Hotel in North Beach, the neighborhood that, fifty years later, would birth another generation of free thinkers: the Beats.[14]

Brown kept in touch with a few of Les Jeunes in the succeeding years, and Bruce Porter was a close friend for the balance of both their lives. Porter would also help Philip Brown in ways he could not yet foresee, bringing art into the lives of some of his most vulnerable patients.

Philip King Brown seemed to be all about work, but his time spent with the Les Jeunes crowd reveals a bohemian side to his character. Many of these men also shared Brown's deep commitment to social issues. Burgess was a prankster but was devoted to the principles of the Boys' Club. Bruce Porter's art helped move forward the Arts and Crafts movement, which went beyond art and into philosophies wedded to respect for the land. Frank Norris took on the corrupt Southern Pacific Railroad in his seminal novel *The Octopus*, which explored how economic forces were crushing individual initiative in the Gilded Age. Philip chose friends with substance—as he would soon do with the woman who became his wife.

Hospital appointments and teaching jobs, ranging from the University of California to the Eye and Ear Hospital, now came his way. Even though he held multiple hospital and university appointments and had his own private practice, the busy Philip King Brown was also expected to make the rounds of the social scene. He appeared in the society pages frequently, and he bumped elbows and conversed with some of San Francisco's biggest names.

Phoebe Hearst's was among them. He got back in touch with her after his postgraduate work, and he returned to his service with the Boys' Club. They intersected in other places too. In 1897 Philip King Brown started running one of the medical clinics at the San Francisco Polyclinic, a dispensary for the poor founded above a stable in the Tenderloin neighborhood in 1888. Polyclinics opened all over the United States in the late nineteenth century so that newly qualified doctors could get postgraduate education and practical experience. There were separate clinics for the various specialties: gynecology; ear, nose, and throat; and internal medicine. Treatment was free, and patients had to pay only for medications.[15]

Phoebe Hearst was a big San Francisco Polyclinic supporter. By the 1890s the place was in better quarters, though still in the Tenderloin district, where it was most needed. Philip Brown's commitment to the polyclinic brought the two of them together at a place where their passions could be realized.

Philip King Brown and Phoebe Hearst corresponded throughout the 1890s. On April 5, 1899, he sent her a letter that sounds like the continuation of a conversation about the number of bad doctors in California. He ended his letter with a very personal paragraph, a liberty he could only have taken had their relationship gone beyond their mutual interest in the Boys' Club. "I always think of you as I have seen you so often, with so many young people about you who seem to belong to you."[16] It was a compliment to her influence. But he may have also been thinking of one young person in particular.

～

On March 8 and 9, 1900, two San Francisco newspapers, the *Call* and the *Chronicle*, published articles about an unexpected wedding. The *Call*'s headline:

"Nuptials of Dr. Brown and Miss Hillyer Surprise Their Friends." The wedding may have been a surprise to San Francisco society, but not to the bride and groom. Philip Brown and Helen Hillyer had met sometime in 1898, and their immediate attraction to each other matched their values and their backgrounds. Not only that: Helen Hillyer's childhood was almost as eventful as Charlotte Brown's.

Helen's parents, Ohio-born Munson Curtis Hillyer and New Jersey native Martha Lowe, came to California via New Orleans and the Isthmus of Panama in 1851. Munson worked for a flour merchant in San Francisco and eventually held an interest in a flour mill on his own. The couple lost a daughter in infancy and then had a son named Frank in 1854, followed by another daughter, Florence, in 1857.

Flour brought home the bacon in the Hillyer household, but Munson was always drawn to mining. During the early 1860s, he spent time in Virginia City, Nevada, the heart of the Comstock silver strike, and he eventually began to deal in mining stocks. He had a Midas touch for finding prosperous mines, just like one of his new friends: George Hearst.

Martha and the children stayed in San Francisco while Munson wandered around Nevada, but tragedy brought him home. In July 1867, thirteen-year-old Frank Hillyer died in an accident with a hunting rifle. The Hillyers struggled along, but in 1869 Munson moved them to Treasure City, in White Pine County, Nevada, where there were new silver strikes. Martha Hillyer, who had always been fragile, found herself pregnant again, and the family returned to San Francisco. Their daughter was born there on July 12, 1871, and named Helen Adelaide.

Helen's sister, Florence, married a San Francisco attorney in 1877. In 1882 Martha became so ill that she had to move to southern California to recuperate, and she entrusted her preteen daughter to the care of Phoebe Hearst, who had become as dear a friend as George Hearst had become to her husband. Helen went to live with Phoebe and George in their suite at the posh Baldwin Hotel in San Francisco, but Helen was very close to her father. Whenever she could, she wanted to be by his side. In 1884 he went to Alaska to investigate new mines, while also serving as a U.S. marshal, and she went with him for a few months. After she returned to San Francisco, she continued her schooling, which by her own admission was hit and miss.

Helen Hillyer's mother died in June 1885. Munson still needed to support himself and his daughter, and he decided to try his luck in Colombian mines, migrating between South America and New York. At their urging, Helen moved to Washington to live with the Hearsts and was under Phoebe's wing (and occasionally back in San Francisco) through the end of the 1880s. Phoebe Hearst's friendship sustained her when her father died in 1889, and Helen then began to accompany Phoebe on many international trips, serving as her hostess, companion, and surrogate daughter.

When Helen Hillyer returned to San Francisco at the end of 1899 after a trip around Europe and the Middle East, there was one person she was most anxious to see. The very night she arrived in the city, her friends begged her to join them for dinner out, but she wanted to sit by the telephone at her sister's house. As she had hoped, it soon rang and Philip King Brown's voice was on the other end.[17]

He was unlike any of the young society men Helen was expected to go out with. Philip Brown was not a flibbertigibbet; he didn't care about sports or spend his free time smoking cigars in men's clubs. He was involved with organizations that were important to Phoebe Hearst, which endeared him to Helen immediately. For his part, he wanted a woman who had just as much substance and depth of character.

Philip and Helen were married in Phoebe's apartments in the Hearst Building in San Francisco on March 7, 1900. After the ceremony, the couple left for a long honeymoon. It would include a visit to some of Philip Brown's friends from Harvard in Boston and then a medical conference in Washington, D.C. But their first stop was beautiful Santa Barbara.

Philip King Brown's cousin Anna S. C. Blake owned a spectacular home in Montecito, a few miles from Santa Barbara. He had been her physician in the last years of her life, and when she died in March 1899, she left Brown her house and a large endowment so that he could turn the estate into a convalescent home or sanitarium. He took on this task willingly but understood the challenges he would face.

It was here, at the place Philip King Brown named Miradero, that the Browns started their married life. And as Helen had no doubt expected, her husband wrote to Phoebe Hearst about his plans just a few weeks after the wedding. "This is a business letter, the kind you used to get from me long ago, only this one is more personal than it used to be," as he said in one early missive.[18]

He asked her to be a Miradero trustee and said that he expected to open the sanitarium in September or October. "If I make the trial & fail, the whole property reverts to the residual heirs, but I shall not fail."[19] The Browns planned to leave for the East on April 3, and on April 2 the property was officially turned over to Philip's care. That same day he also he received a letter from Phoebe in which she agreed to be a trustee. His gratitude was unbounded, and in the letters he would send to Phoebe throughout the honeymoon, the previously reserved Philip King Brown would speak with eloquence and humility about his love for Helen and his sure knowledge that his life had really begun.

The couple returned to San Francisco in the summer and moved in with Philip's parents for a few months before getting their own place just a block away. Their happiness increased on February 6, 1901, with the birth of their first child, a boy called Hillyer Blake Brown. Over the next year, Philip King Brown saw to his practice and gave papers at medical meetings, and he and Helen went to small private dinners and big social events. On April 18, 1902, Philip and Helen welcomed their second son, Harrison Cabot, known always as Cabot.

Philip King Brown was destined to be surrounded by strong women, and the first and most influential was of course his mother, Charlotte. Even as her children's careers and personal lives took off and Dr. Charlotte Brown entered her fifties, she did not slow down. Now a stout matron with silver-white hair, she was sought out to be the patroness for a variety of new organizations, which were arriving at increasing speed as the new century opened.

Charlotte, Henry, and Adelaide Brown lived just a block from fashionable Van Ness Avenue, the wide thoroughfare that separated the financial district from the bright, large homes of San Francisco's wealthy on its west side. Though she seemed to have unlimited energy, Charlotte Brown had started taking time off now and then for her health. In 1893 she went to Miradero to rest for a few weeks, and in 1894 and 1898 she spent time at Vichy Springs in Ukiah, a few hours north of San Francisco, enjoying the benefits of its natural mineral waters.

She may have needed the time away for another reason, because her husband, Henry, was involved in yet another scandal. Rumors had bubbled around town that he was paying attention to a Louisa Hislop, wife of George Hislop, the agent for a local manufacturer. In November 1902 the couple split up but stayed in separate households within their large home near Golden Gate Park. In December 1903 Louisa filed for a divorce, citing Hislop's infidelity with a woman named Violette. He turned around in February 1904 and sued Henry Brown for alienation of affection, claiming that he had given Louisa money, jewelry, furniture, and fine dresses for more than a year.

George then went even further and said that Louisa had moved out and was living with Henry Brown in a house on Clayton Street, a few blocks away from their home. As with many scandals of the period, and especially since all official records were lost in the fires of 1906, there is no way to know the truth. Records that do exist make it clear that Henry Brown lived with his wife and daughter, but whether he owned a house on Clayton is an open question. What we do know is that Henry settled with George Hislop. He offered him a "nominal sum" to avoid notoriety and the suit was then dismissed.[20]

In April 1904 Dr. Charlotte Brown was fifty-seven years old, and her dark eyes still sparkled as she practiced her profession. But she was tired, and early that month she developed an intestinal problem that required emergency surgery at the Adler Sanatorium near her home. To everyone's shock, she did not survive the operation. She died on April 19.

No letters or diaries survive to tell us how Philip King Brown felt about the loss of the woman whose example inspired him into medicine. As a doctor, he understood more than most how quickly simple illness could turn into tragedy. So he mourned with his sisters and his mother's many friends and then got back to work and to living. He and Helen bought a large home on Van Ness Avenue in 1905, and the household was increased again on June 22 with the birth of their first girl. They had no trouble deciding what to name her: Phoebe Hearst Brown.

On April 17, 1906, they went to sleep having every reason to believe that their lives would continue to be as happy as they had been since their wedding day. Philip Brown had a fulfilling career, Helen gave her time to charities and the suffrage movement, they would likely have more children, and their financial situation was solid. They closed their eyes that night secure in the knowledge that the following day would be as full of blessings and opportunities as the one now passing into the quiet, starry night.

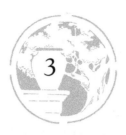

3

CONSUMED

THE GREAT SAN FRANCISCO EARTHQUAKE was actually two quakes—for the first couple of minutes anyway.

At 5:12 A.M. on Wednesday, April 18, 1906, residents were shaken by a strong temblor that lasted only a few seconds. Blasé natives mostly turned over and went back to sleep, if the quake even woke them at all. But then came the second one, which lasted a minute or more (depending on who was doing the reporting). That doesn't sound like a long time, but when the unyielding earth suddenly has a life of its own, it can be an eternity.

Your experience of the quake depended on where you were. Some people, still in their homes, said the shocks went back and forth and then twisted, knocking them out of bed or down stairwells. Men and women walking outdoors couldn't keep on their feet because the pavement was heaving like the sea. Cobblestones bounced like marbles in a bag. Later, many who lived through it said the sensation was like a terrier shaking a rat. Others called the quake a wiggle. (A few probably shared my native Californian experience with earthquakes: feeling like a bug in a jar being shaken by a particularly vicious five-year-old.)

After the earth threw them up in the air or pulled them down to the ground, San Franciscans saw sights they didn't have words for. Streetcar tracks came unbolted and snapped vertically off the ground, waving in the air like creatures trying to crawl out of the chasms that opened underneath them. Multifloored buildings pancaked to the street. Roofs were where cellars should have been.

And everywhere were people in nightclothes, or partially dressed, holding household objects or each other, staring, unable to speak. After a great and horrible silence, the groans and screams began—from the wounded who staggered through crumbled doorways and the terrified trapped under bricks and boards. Doctors and nurses left their own homes and ran to city hospitals to help the streams of wounded, and within hours boats brought medical personnel and supplies from outlying counties.

Fires had started sprouting within minutes of the first shakes, and with terrifying speed fifty separate blazes soon blanketed the city. Many converged into gigantic roaring firestorms. Firefighters were shocked to realize that the earthquake had shattered many of the city's water mains, and broken gas lines were fueling the fires. Water pumped from the bay helped quell the flames near the waterfront, but the worst hit areas farther inland were under fiery siege.

The military then made a fateful decision: it would dynamite homes along Van Ness Avenue. This would create a firebreak, halting the flames from spreading farther west. In theory this was a good idea, but with so many different kinds of explosives being used, and little or no water handy to put out the additional fires they started, the dynamiting caused more problems than it solved. The fire did stop at Van Ness, though whether it was because the exploded structures gave the flames no more fuel or simply because the street was so wide is still an open question. The fires were finally extinguished after three terrible days.

Meanwhile, the army set up refugee camps in Golden Gate Park and other public spaces throughout the city. There were also unofficial encampments on streets and in parks, which worried officials concerned about disease. Within a few months the army also built five thousand tiny wooden houses for refugees; some lived there for the next two full years. The luckiest survivors had family and friends to take them in, but many more didn't have this option. Relief systems were scarce and disorganized, but politicians, charity workers, and military authorities worked together within and outside official channels after the disaster.

Despite losing their home and Philip losing his office, the Browns took over an abandoned house belonging to a friend and opened a relief station, registration bureau, and bureau of information, so that people could find their lost relatives. Philip King Brown's sister Adelaide started up an emergency medical clinic in the house and managed to strong-arm friends into loaning her their cars so she could transport the injured from nearby crowded hospitals or tent encampments. Once the wounded were stabilized, volunteers drove them to the ferry so they could get to relatives or hospitals outside San Francisco. Adelaide Brown also found ranchers in nearby counties who sent her milk and eggs.

The Browns' bureau and clinic stayed open for ten days, and then the Presidio medical department, the San Francisco Board of Health, and other organizations officially took charge of relief efforts. Philip and Helen Brown rented a furnished house about a mile west of their Van Ness Avenue home, moved in their children, and got their lives and careers going again.[1]

By the summer of 1906, Philip King Brown was back into his routine and had cobbled together an office in the family's rented house. He spoke at medical conferences and published papers throughout the rest of 1907. He and Helen decided to buy a plot of land and build a new home, and they started looking around for a larger rented place to live in while it was under construction. The year ended quietly, which was a relief after the physical and emotional shocks of 1906. But the previous eighteen months had created a shift in Brown's focus as a doctor, and as 1908 opened, his name and his work were entwined with a new threat to San Francisco's residents.

∾

Despite everyone's best efforts, once the original crisis was over, disease stalked the post-earthquake city. Both sick and healthy people were crammed together in tent cities or in houses now sheltering multiple families. The deadliest threat was typhoid, which erupted quickly throughout the city. Plague soon followed, carried by the rats now racing through the streets after being burned out of their hidey-holes. Doctors scrambled to contain these threats, but they were not brought under control until more rigid inspections in the refugee camps led to cleaner latrines and living areas, and until water mains were repaired, bringing drinkable water into rebuilt homes.

In January 1908 Bay Area newspapers ran articles about an important conference planned for the fall: the International Congress on Tuberculosis. Every state in the Union was choosing representatives to go to the Washington, D.C., meeting, and Philip King Brown was part of the California contingent.[2] He had quietly turned into a tuberculosis expert, but his voice would be louder as the year progressed.

Tuberculosis is a disease of the unsanitary and the crowded, and it begins with something small but deadly: a bacillus, or bacterium, a single-celled organism that a person either inhales in air particles or ingests with something infected, such as milk. (Cows can carry tuberculosis.) TB can affect any part of the body, but the lungs are especially vulnerable.

If a person is healthy and her immune system is not compromised in any way, her body can fight off the invasion. However, if the person has other underlying conditions, the bacillus takes up residence in the lungs. It starts to multiply, and the resulting bacilli form tubercles, which are swellings or nodules attached to organs (think tuber, or something resembling a small potato). These eat away at lung tissue, creating gaping cavities, blocking the body's ability to process oxygen. The infected person coughs all the time, bringing up sputum, or phlegm, that teems with bacilli. These become airborne, and when they do, they spread out to attach themselves to the next victim. TB transmission is easy, which is why it is so terrifying.

Tuberculosis, known for centuries as consumption, is found all over the world and has been part of American life since the first Europeans landed. Starting in the colonial period, doctors and society at large thought the disease was hereditary rather than contagious. There was even a "TB type": thin-limbed, hollow-chested, pale, and weak. Poets, writers, and other overly sensitive souls were thought to be particularly susceptible to consumption.

The name itself comes from what the disease brought to the body: weight loss, weakness, coughing, bringing up blood, and shortness of breath, signs that meant sufferers were not long for this world. They looked eaten alive from the inside; consumed. And no treatment to relieve their suffering existed. People simply stayed home, lay in their beds or on couches, and literally wasted away, all the while not knowing how dangerous they were to their families, friends, and communities.

The first small movements toward identifying and finding a treatment for TB came out of Germany in the mid-nineteenth century. Two doctors, Hermann Brehmer and Peter Dettweiler, thought that people with consumption should be separated from society and medically supervised in institutions devoted specifically to their care. These were generally in the mountains, where the air was considered purer.[3]

In 1882 consumptive life was changed forever. Dr. Robert Koch, an 1866 graduate of the University of Göttingen, had dedicated his professional life to bacteriology and made breakthroughs in the study of diseases such as anthrax. He then turned his attention to consumption. He was sure it was infectious and not hereditary, but no one had been able to identify the organism responsible. After years of work, he announced to the Physiological Society of Berlin that he had isolated the tubercle bacillus, the bacterium responsible for consumption. The horror now had a physical cause and, soon, a new name: tuberculosis.

Even as Koch was making his discovery, doctors in the United States were trying to find ways to cure TB or, even better, to keep people from getting it in the first place. They knew that crowded, urban conditions were the perfect petri dish for tuberculosis, and both they and their patients began to look to the unsullied air and open spaces of the Southwest, the Rocky Mountains, and especially California for treatment. Rather than rest, the vigorous and healthy life of the rugged West became the goal (for men, mostly), and many people who did conquer the disease this way wrote glowing letters and pamphlets about their experiences.

Former consumptives weren't the only boosters. Many doctors were confident that the geography and climate of the West was the key to health. Their conclusions were not really very scientific, and people kept dying from TB whether they lived and breathed in the mountains of Colorado or the deserts of Arizona. Doctors were sometimes TB patients themselves, and they frequently found that their long-held beliefs did not hold true when they were doing the coughing. But one physician ended up not only winning his personal battle against TB but also finding a way to heal others.

Edward Livingston Trudeau was born in New York City in 1848, spent his youth with his family in Paris, and went to Columbia University after returning to the States. He planned to go into the U.S. Naval Academy at Annapolis until he learned that his beloved older brother, James, had contracted tuberculosis. Trudeau dropped everything to stay home and take care of him, but James lasted only three months. In his grief, Trudeau upended the course of his life. He decided to become a doctor instead of a naval officer, and enrolled in the College of Physicians and Surgeons in New York. He graduated in 1871 and married fellow New Yorker Charlotte Beare the same year. But in 1872 he was shocked to learn that he had developed consumption himself, contracted by nursing his suffering brother.

His own doctor prescribed time out of doors, and after spending months riding horseback in South Carolina, Trudeau returned home as sick as ever. A friend suggested that they go to the Adirondacks, and in June 1873, fully expecting that it would be the last trip of his life, Trudeau left his wife and their two children behind and dragged himself into the mountains, staying at a small hotel that catered to hunters and outdoorsmen. By the end of the summer he was a different man: heavier, tanned, and full of energy. He went home elated at his recovery, but once he was back in his city routine, his symptoms came back.

After another attempt at the outdoor life in Minnesota, he returned to the Adirondacks in June 1874, this time with his family. He stayed throughout the winter and was surprised to see how well he felt, even outdoors in the harsh north country weather. He decided to move permanently to the mountains he had come to love and count on. He set up a medical practice among the lumber-jacks and other working people who lived in the area.

He read in medical journals about how Drs. Brehmer and Dettweiler were treating consumptives in supervised institutions and saw how his own cure mirrored some of their methods. Then he read about Koch's discovery of the tubercle bacillus, and he began to replicate Koch's experiments after teaching himself how to use a microscope. He knew that he had the knowledge and the means to combine everything he knew about the disease to offer a cure to the hopeless.

He realized that the bacillus, even while invading the lungs, could be combated by increasing the vitality of the body itself through good hygiene, the right amount of fresh air, and the most nutritious food. "How" was more important than "where."

Trudeau had just invented the tuberculosis rest cure. Other doctors took notice.

The doctor and his family now lived in Saranac Lake, New York, and in 1885 he decided to create an institution where TB sufferers could take the cure under his guidance. He offered free medical treatment to the poor from all over the region, lodging them in individual "cure cottages" for minimal rent. He named his new venture the Adirondack Cottage Sanitarium, making it the first tuberculosis sanatorium in America and the model for the many others which were soon to come.[4]

Although Trudeau used the term *sanitarium* for the name of his institution, *sanatorium* was a more accurate description for places that treated patients with tuberculosis.

A sanitarium was where you spent a few days or weeks to regain your general health if you were nervous, weak, or drying out (the word came from the Latin *sanitas*, meaning "health"). Some sanitariums were built near mineral springs, and guests would drink foul-tasting mineral waters to boost their vitality or to cure various ailments. A sanitarium was, in a way, a more rigorous version of a modern spa.

On the other hand, you went to a sanatorium if you had a specific illness like tuberculosis (from the Latin *sanare*, meaning "to cure" or "to heal"). You usually stayed there until you were cured. Or dead. A sanatorium was serious business, and you had a very serious illness if that was the word above the entrance.

However, no one was ever "cured" at a tuberculosis sanatorium. Although doctors sometimes used that word, they always wrote "apparently" in front of

it. People could conquer active TB in their bodies if they faithfully followed the
methods that Trudeau experimented with and then put in place at his sanatorium. If caught in its early stages, TB could be slowed and even halted.

If a patient got rest, good nutrition to build up the immune system, and
lots of fresh air, cells known as macrophages formed in the lungs, walling off
the bacilli into a type of scar tissue. When this process was successful, the
bacilli stopped growing and the sufferer was no longer contagious. By living
without stress, staying healthy, and keeping chronic diseases in check, people
who once had tuberculosis could live for decades. However, if the situation
changed, the scars could open up and spread the bacilli again. There was
no cure for TB then—simply an arrest of symptoms. Tuberculosis was a life
sentence.

With everyone packed together after the earthquake, doctors such as Philip
King Brown were worried about TB transmission and convinced the administrators at San Francisco's City and County Hospital to open a tuberculosis ward.
Located in the sparsely populated working-class district called Potrero Hill,
south of downtown, the hospital was a rickety, substandard structure whose
beds were filled mostly with the poor. Brown was an attending physician there,
and he wasn't happy about the conditions the patients had to live in. He was even
more worried about all the pulmonary cases showing up after the earthquake.
City and County's response was to open a "tubercular colony" on the hospital's
grounds. The administration erected tents for patients and doctors, and built a
kitchen, lavatory, and dining areas. It was very sanatorium-like, but there wasn't
room for everyone who needed it.

In August 1908 Philip King Brown and a number of other doctors asked the
city's board of supervisors for extra money to treat the hospital's acute cases.
He was blunt about how bad things were. There was not one curable case in
the TB ward, he said, because there weren't enough doctors or proper facilities
to fight the disease. He made a motion, which was passed, that patients with
critical cases of TB be separated from those with incipient cases. He also got an
agreement to put the women in a ward separate from the men.[5]

He was starting to think like Trudeau.

City and County was completely demolished later that year, and a new hospital, now Zuckerberg San Francisco General, was built in its place. But the new
hospital had fewer beds for TB patients, and local doctors knew this was a crisis

that needed addressing. Philip King Brown had already been thinking about the problem and had a few solutions up his sleeve.

Earlier that year he had published an article in *Journal of the Outdoor Life*, organ of the newly formed National Tuberculosis Association. Titled "Outdoor Life in California," it looked at first glance like a PR man's pamphlet about the land of flowers, fruit, and sunshine. But Brown got right to the point in the first paragraph, saying that the state's climate made California the perfect health resort for consumptives.

He then outlined his two-pronged approach to fighting tuberculosis: (1) living outdoors was the best preventive against TB and the best hope for recovery; (2) the outdoor life was essential in California because there were no public institutions where TB patients could take the cure. Living in the out-of-doors was better than living in close, indoor quarters, where dust and dirt from San Francisco's ongoing rebuilding found places to settle, making breathing even harder.[6]

Philip King Brown used his article to agitate for more municipal sanatoria, pointing out that the only institutions being built to treat TB in California were privately funded and managed, and few in number. He specifically mentioned Barlow Sanatorium in Los Angeles, which was opened in 1902 near where Dodger Stadium is today. Brown knew its founder, W. Jarvis Barlow, and he and Helen visited Dr. and Mrs. Barlow in the summer of 1906 to see how the sanatorium worked. Even then, he knew that TB was going to be a big problem for San Francisco. But until more city and county institutions were opened for business, the important thing was to keep people from getting it in the first place. And the best way to make this happen was to convince the vulnerable to spend as much time outdoors as possible.

Philip King Brown grabbed any opportunity to spread his word about outdoor life and the need for more sanatorium beds for TB patients, even before he went to Washington to attend the international TB conference. He was single-minded on this topic, but he never neglected his other patients, his family, or his social obligations. Whenever they could, he and Helen visited Phoebe Hearst. They also watched their new house being built on a cliff overlooking the Golden Gate. But his commitment to TB prevention was always there, and he had found a way to bridge the topics of education, self-responsibility, and prevention to reach the greatest number of people.

He started a class.

He had the perfect captive audience and the perfect place for his TB classroom at the San Francisco Polyclinic. Like Phoebe Hearst, he thought education could take many forms. He was convinced that if people knew enough about TB prevention, they could keep themselves healthy and keep the disease from decimating their families and neighborhoods. They could use the same lessons to keep TB from coming back if they were lucky enough to recover from it in the first place.

He started talking to those who came to the polyclinic for treatment and soon had regular attendees for his classes. Typically, Brown or another doctor, a nurse, and a social worker met with each individual "student," who was weighed and interviewed about the number of hours they spent outdoors, the size and frequency of their meals, how much sputum they coughed up, and so on.

The staff also taught people how to spend time out of doors even if they lived in a boardinghouse or apartment. They could build outdoor sleeping platforms or enclose porches with screens so they could sleep all night in the open air. Fire escapes were also excellent sleeping areas in good weather, and so were roofs. Lacking a porch or a fire escape was no excuse for living in stuffy quarters, because everyone could leave their windows open.

All this exposure to air was a difficult mental and cultural shift, however. Despite the common understanding about the germ theory of medicine and the ways that TB was spread, many people still thought you could catch tuberculosis by catching a chill. Drafts had been blamed for all kinds of illnesses for centuries, and Philip King Brown knew he had to shatter this belief before anyone could be helped.

The polyclinic also helped the attendees at the TB class in ways that went beyond the medical; the doctors and other staff members bought milk and eggs for patients and sometimes found charities that would take in children while one or the other parent was taking the rest cure at home.

The class wasn't cheap to run, but local philanthropists donated enough money to keep it going after the first year and well into a second. Dr. Brown saw real improvement in the patients who followed his advice. But it didn't work for everyone. In September 1909 he published an article in the *Merchants Association Review* titled "Tuberculosis Class Work in the San Francisco Polyclinic," which spelled out where the greatest need really was. He saw favorable results in early cases of TB in the students—but only among men. And he knew exactly why.

"The opportunities that are open to women are distinctly against them, not only being conducive to the acquiring of tuberculosis, but offering a minimum of opportunity for recovery under the present conditions. . . . The outdoor occupations which are plentiful for men in California are hardly open to them at all and . . . when they acquire a tubercular lung infection they are very apt to go steadily down hill."[7]

Philip King Brown felt that all women were at great risk for TB, but the ones he worried about the most were those his mother often treated and talked about, the ones who left their homes every day to work in factories, schoolrooms, offices, and shops. They were the "working girls" of San Francisco.

~

America's women had been working in textile factories and light industry since the early nineteenth century, but their numbers swelled in the years after the Civil War. Some women worked because their families had lost their livelihoods and their property in the war, or the menfolk were dead or injured beyond recovery. The 1860s and 1870s were also a time of unprecedented invention and innovation; new products like the typewriter, paper dress patterns, roller skates, linoleum, the telephone, and the lightbulb needed factories to produce them and consumers to use them. The market for ready-to-wear clothing also exploded, and factories hired thousands of women, who applied their home sewing skills to mass production.[8]

Factory work brought many young rural women into cities. Though they worked long hours and lived in crowded conditions, for some the freedom to earn their own living and the pleasures they could now pay for were more than compensation for the hardships. Office jobs were also a new avenue of work, and the women who managed the newfangled machines in men's offices were themselves called typewriters. The labor was lighter, but the hours were as long and supervision as strict—and as sexually overbearing—as they were in factories, disillusioning young women quickly. Traditional jobs such as teaching and domestic service, which could be even more physically tiring than working a sewing machine, were not the avenue to an independent life.[9]

But sometimes a young woman's job meant food on the table for her elderly parents, and a personal life took second place to survival. Married women worked outside the home only out of the deepest urgency; perhaps their husbands were sick or couldn't find work. Sometimes they were divorced or widowed. If they had children, they were lucky if they had someone to watch the kids during the workday, but they had to fulfill all their motherly duties once they got home. Philip King Brown would later call these "thousands of little unavoidable cares."[10] And even if they stayed at home with the children while their husbands went off to work, women might labor to make artificial flowers, take in washing and sewing, or cook and clean for the rough and unruly men who sometimes boarded in their homes. The working class lived in a spiral of low wages and the constant threat of unemployment that kept the middle class within view but never within reach.

In the 1870s San Francisco experienced a boom in industrial production thanks in part to its links to the transcontinental railroad. Clothing and boot manufacturing and cigar making were the three largest employers by 1880, and many women found jobs sewing clothes and rolling cigars up to and beyond the turn of the century.[11]

After its transient gold rush youth, San Francisco was now a place for families. Families needed consumer goods and their children needed teachers, and the city's prosperity created a ripple effect of industry that gave wage-earning women many opportunities for employment. Old and new monied households also required laundries, restaurants, beauty parlors, and domestic servants. An abbreviated list of the types of jobs women held in San Francisco in 1910 (as found in the city directory) is only a partial picture of how widespread their labor was: teacher, garment worker, bookbinder, cashier, janitor, stenographer, bookkeeper, telephone operator, department store clerk, grocery store owner, servant, boardinghouse owner.

Here, as in other cities, a job meant something different to every woman. But they all took a physical toll. Telephone operators sat all day reaching and stretching to push phone jacks into a switchboard, sometimes fielding two hundred to three hundred calls per hour. They were under constant supervision by male floor walkers, were not allowed to talk to each other, and could use the bathroom only at scheduled times.

Department store clerks had the opposite problem: they were on their feet all day, which caused pain anywhere their bodies were vulnerable. During inventory season the hours were longer, and many women fainted from exhaustion. They also couldn't use the toilets when they needed to, and many women developed lifelong kidney trouble.[12]

The women who worked at sewing machines almost had to become machines themselves. After the turn of the century, some industrial equipment moved at forty-four hundred stitches a minute, and women had to watch the needle "as a cat watches a mouse hole," in the words of one 1905 *San Francisco Call* article. "By reason of the intolerable speed of the best new sewing machines, operatives wear out and break down if they do not marry out of the trade at an early age. In a tragically large number of cases they do both."[13]

The workplace itself could be as bad as the job duties. Philip King Brown put this concept succinctly in his 1909 "Tuberculosis Class Work" article: "As laundry-workers, dressmakers, clerks, factory-workers, inner-office workers, they are where the most unsanitary conditions in business life are found."[14] Factories were poorly ventilated and even more poorly lit. Hallways and exits might not have any lighting at all. At the end of the workday, tired women heading home often fell down stairwells that were as dark as the early winter nights. Factories of all kinds kept windows closed, causing women to breathe in everything from cotton lint to toxic fumes.

The home life of San Francisco's working-class women and their families added to their daily stress. Single women lived in boardinghouses or shared rooms in cheaply built residential hotels. These had no meal plans, so paying for restaurant food was an added expense. Married women and their families often lived in these places too, because the rooms were cheaper than apartment rentals. Single women who lived in boardinghouses could pay to eat their meals with the other roomers or pay less and find food elsewhere. Or they could lodge with a family and eat at their table.[15]

Women who had grown up in crowded homes with siblings didn't have a problem living in similar situations with strangers—though they did have their standards when it came to finding roommates. In 1905 a young woman placed an ad in the *San Francisco Call*: "WANTED—By respectable, refined working-girl, roommate, to share expenses in a large, comfortably furnished room with housekeeping privileges; centrally located; lady working in office or store preferred; object economy and companionship."[16]

Laborers often chose hotels, flats, or boardinghouses because they were close to the factories and offices where they worked, which saved on the cost of public transportation. These were not the pick of the housing crop though. Multifamily residences tended to be dark, they had poor ventilation and plumbing, and large families or groups of roommates had to share very small spaces. Illness stalked both the home and workplace, and of the many germy dangers that women faced, tuberculosis was the most common. It was so ubiquitous that it was sometimes called a "house disease."[17]

The events of 1906 made a mockery of the word *choice*. The fire had wiped out buildings of all kinds in the working-class and industrial districts south of Market Street. Finding housing became less about options and more about availability, however short-term. Some people could only find living quarters far away from where they worked. And for others, jobs weren't even there anymore.

But laborers who persevered in the city eventually found their way back to normalcy, even if that meant returning to the same living and working conditions they had before April 18.

Men with a vested interest in bringing business back to the city referred to the disaster as "the fire" and not "the earthquake." Fires were accidents that could be prevented in the future; acts of God were not, and their hope was that people and companies would not be scared away from the new San Francisco. But to the city's working class, these nouns meant nothing.

PROGRESSIVES

PHILIP KING BROWN KNEW how burdened wage-earning women were, not only because of what he saw in his own practice but from observing and talking with his mother.

From the day in 1874 when Dr. Charlotte Brown started her own career, women had been her sole concern. She was a big supporter of the new Young Women's Christian Association, for example, and was especially interested in the lunchroom the YWCA opened in 1891 for women who worked in factories in the South of Market industrial district. She knew that young women, in their newly independent working lives, sometimes spent their meager extra pennies on fripperies instead of food. That was a downward path to certain disease.

In April 1896 Dr. Charlotte Brown addressed the annual meeting of the Medical Society of the State of California on the topic "The Health of Our Girls," which was later reprinted as a pamphlet. She thought that young women were not eating well (a particular worry) and not getting enough rest. But even worse, the process of turning active girls into sedate women was just as dangerous for their long-term health. Once they reached adolescence, play was put aside, as "the girl ceases to romp and puts on the dignity of the young woman."[1] This led to a lifetime of inactivity and potential for illness. So Charlotte encouraged local philanthropists to fund gymnastic fields and school administrators to give girls training in physical, manual, and domestic science. Education and activity: that's how you create healthy women, and it didn't matter if they wanted to be mothers or doctors.

Working women got the Charlotte Brown treatment too. In 1901, when women in San Francisco applied to be "hello girls" (telephone operators), they needed to pass a rigorous medical exam. Dr. Brown volunteered to do the examinations, and this was reported with glee in a 1901 article in the *San Francisco*

Call, illustrated with a hilarious caricature of a bespectacled, white-haired Charlotte. "When a telephone 'rooky' hands in her application with a certificate from Mrs. Dr. Brown securely pinned to it she can be sure that she is physically sound from the soles of her feet to the crown of her head."[2] Charlotte took her duties seriously, and when she found woman who were in danger of getting sick or were sick already, she took this opportunity to educate them.

Philip King Brown was seeing a lot of unhealthy women coming into his office, and they were the same type of working women his mother had always cared for. So many of them had tuberculosis, and so many couldn't or wouldn't alter their lives to get better at home. They needed sanatorium care, but there was no place for them to go. Recalling his mother's solution to the desperate medical needs of poor mothers and children, Dr. Brown came to a decision. He would have to build a sanatorium himself.

Just for women.

∼

Philip King Brown wasn't the first doctor to have this idea, not even in California. In 1910 an English physician named George Martyn opened a sanatorium in the Pasadena foothills for women in the early stages of tuberculosis. The following year, a quarter century after Edward Trudeau opened his Adirondack sanatorium, the National Association for the Study and Prevention of Tuberculosis published a directory containing a list of more than four hundred sanatoria across forty-four states. Some were privately owned and funded; others were run by cities and counties, religious orders, and fraternal organizations. However, the 1911 directory showed only eleven institutions for tubercular women exclusively: four in Massachusetts, four in New York, one in Ohio, one in Pennsylvania, and the Martyn Sanatorium in California.

New York City had St. George's Roof Camp for Tuberculosis, and Toledo had the Thalian Fresh Air Camp. These places were exactly what they sound like: rustic and camp-like, intended to mimic the outdoor life of the Adirondacks, housing people in large tents or a few permanent structures.

Other TB refuges were charitable institutions that predated the sanatorium movement but now took TB patients as part of their mission—the House of the Good Samaritan in Boston, for example (for white women only), and the Channing Home in Boston. The Syracuse Hospital in New York added a TB wing in 1909 just for women. And the Mount St. Michael's Sanatorium in Reading, Pennsylvania, was for Catholic nuns only.

Of all the women-only TB institutions in the TB directory, Stony Wold in Lake Kushaqua, New York; the Sharon Sanatorium in Sharon, Massachusetts; and the Martyn Sanatorium in Pasadena were the closest in mission and treatment to what Philip King Brown had in mind. When his sanatorium opened, it would be the first of its kind in northern California and only the second one exclusively for women in the entire West.

The Bay Area already had a few tuberculosis sanatoria. Close by were the California Sanatorium for the Treatment of Tuberculosis in Belmont, south of San Francisco; the Diggins Sanatorium in San Francisco; and the TB wards of City and County Hospital in San Francisco. But these took in both men and women, which meant they were treated the same way, which really meant that the women were cared for as if they were men—or worse, just tubercular bodies. These places were overcrowded, the staffs were overburdened, and no one was teaching the patients how to get well and how to stay that way.[3]

What Dr. Brown wanted was a sanatorium built along the philosophical lines of the San Francisco Polyclinic class but aimed at women alone, because their need was greater. With his own sanatorium, he could not only teach them; he could also learn from them. Once he made his decision, he jumped into his project with the same fervor he'd seen in his mother when she plotted and planned her own hospital. He may have been just a young boy then, but the example and the activity were not lost on him.

Before he could build his sanatorium, Dr. Brown needed land to put it on. Thanks to the web of his social and philanthropic acquaintances, a millionaire named Henry Bothin was about to come into his orbit and solve this problem.

Born in Wisconsin in 1853, farm boy Henry moved to San Francisco at the age of eighteen to find a better way to make a living. He began in the tea and spice importing trade and then moved into manufacturing iron and steel in San Francisco's South of Market industrial district. He also amassed significant real estate in the city and northward, in Marin County, a quiet agricultural, ranching, and dairy region easily accessed by the ferry boats that crossed San Francisco Bay. By the end of the 1880s he was wealthy and connected, and after 1900 he turned his interests and his fortune to philanthropy. An early beneficiary was a nurse named Elizabeth Ashe.

She was born into the family for whom the city of Asheville, North Carolina, was named. She was also the niece of Civil War admiral David Farragut, responsible for the Union victory at the Battle of Mobile Bay and famous for the wartime rallying cry "Damn the torpedoes! Full speed ahead!" In 1869 her parents, Richard Porter Ashe and Caroline Loyall, were living in Stockton, where they had considerable property, and she was born in that Central Valley town, the last of seven children. She grew up in San Francisco, and although she was from a social class that enjoyed money, position, and leisure, she yearned for something more than a life of parties and dances, much like Helen Hillyer. Her compassionate mother had also raised her to think of and act for the poor whenever possible. As she entered adulthood, Elizabeth turned her sights toward social service.

In 1888 she met Alice Griffith, a like-minded and well-off native Californian four years her senior. They taught Sunday School classes at Grace Cathedral to the poor children from the nearby Telegraph Hill area, in today's North Beach district. In 1890 they realized the children needed more than religious instruction, so they formed an organization called the Willing Circle and began to offer sewing, housekeeping, and other practical classes to their pupils. These were so well attended that the two young women changed the name of their group to the City Front Association and began to teach in the neighborhoods where the children and their parents lived.

When the Spanish-American War brought wounded men to the city, Elizabeth helped organize an ambulance corps. She was moved and horrified by the condition of the men, who were battered by war and prey to terrible infectious diseases. She knew that if she continued to work with the poor—where she saw some of the same illnesses, such as typhoid—she would need to know a lot more about medicine. So in 1899, at the age of thirty, Elizabeth decided to enter nursing school. She moved to New York to get her training at Presbyterian Hospital, spending three years in rigorous study. After graduating in 1902, she stayed in the city and worked with Lillian Wald, founder of the famed Henry Street Settlement.

Settlements were an English invention dating to the mid-1880s, and by the end of the decade they were found in nearly every major city in the United States. They were a response to the horrors dealt to the working poor by the industrial age, and the reformers who created them had a unique way of doing their work: they moved into homes in the poorest sections of large cities such as Boston and New York. Hull House in Chicago, founded by future Nobel Peace Prize recipient Jane Addams, was the first and the most famous of all settlement houses. Lillian Wald's Henry Street had opened its doors in 1893.

In these community hubs, residents and volunteer workers gave classes and opened medical clinics for their neighbors. The education they offered ranged

from baby care to English literacy. The houses were definitely tools of assimi-
lation for the exploding immigrant population, but the overarching goal was
to lift the poor metaphorically and literally off the street. Women were in the
majority as settlement workers and gained as much personal and spiritual satisfaction as the people they helped. They also learned political activism, and the
settlement movement was a force for deep social and cultural reform.

As she observed and participated in the daily routine at Henry Street, Elizabeth began to realize how it could be adapted once she got home to San Francisco
later in 1902. Her friend Alice agreed with her, in December the two women
opened the Telegraph Hill Neighborhood House in their old stomping grounds
of North Beach. It had a kitchen garden, sewing school, first aid room, and San
Francisco's first visiting nurses, who went into the homes of the poor to dispense
medicine, deliver babies, and check on the welfare of everyone they could.

By 1903 the Neighborhood House had a dispensary and clinic, and Elizabeth's social circle came through with money and household goods. A wealthy
woman in Marin County named Harriette Kittle had a cottage on her property
in the village of Ross, then as now a haven for the well-to-do, and she knew
Elizabeth Ashe. Kittle let Elizabeth bring children from Telegraph Hill to the
cottage so they could have a country outing, which she did via regular trips on
the bay ferries.

Henry Bothin and his wife, Ellen, also had property in Ross, and he wanted
to buy up more land—not to live on but to put to some sort of philanthropic
use. In February 1903 Bothin bought more than one thousand acres near the
West Marin town of Fairfax, on a railroad line connecting the coast and rich
valleys, carrying lumber and local dairy and farm products to the San Francisco
ferries. The site was an old land grant left over from California's Mexican era
and actually belonged to Phoebe Hearst.

Rich soil, a water supply, and easy access to the bay meant that the property was a commercial gold mine, and rumors about Henry Bothin's possible
plans for the spot began to bubble around Marin; a vacation home, subdividing
the spot for development, and starting a water company were among the top
speculations. But Henry had other ideas, which quickly coalesced after he met
Elizabeth one summer day on the bay ferry.

She was returning to San Francisco, holding on her lap a polio-stricken boy
she had taken to Ross for some time in the sun. Henry was on the same boat,
watching her, and came over to introduce himself and ask about the child. She
explained who she was, told him about the Neighborhood House, and told how

Kittle's cottage was a lifeline for the few children she could take there when she had time. He listened thoughtfully, and they stayed in touch after they parted ways in the city. She later found out that Henry's son had died of polio, which explained his initial interest. But it was Elizabeth's vision that really touched him, and within a few weeks he offered to give her acreage on the old Hearst land near Fairfax so she could create a true country home for city children.

It took nearly two years to realize the project, but in the spring of 1905, a renovated farmhouse on the property was ready to receive its first guests. Twelve children arrived on June 1 to the newly christened Hill Farm, which stayed open into the late fall while the weather remained warm. It closed for the winter and then reopened a week after the earthquake and fire, ultimately becoming an adjunct refugee camp for more than 250 displaced people.

Hill Farm prospered, and doctors, nurses, and teachers volunteered many hours there. Henry and Ellen took a special interest in the place, and in June 1909 they helped sponsor a fund-raiser. By early 1910 Henry was so impressed with the work Elizabeth was doing that he wanted to incorporate the farm as some sort of convalescent association. He also told Elizabeth he was willing to give her more land, and while visiting her at Hill Farm one day, he asked how much more she needed. She reportedly looked up at the surrounding hills and told him she wanted as much land as she could see. That turned out to be 122 additional acres, which Henry turned over without blinking.

Henry signed the final incorporation papers on September 23, 1910. The organization's official name was the Bothin Convalescent Home, which reflected Elizabeth's desire to make Hill Farm not just a country getaway but a place where children could go to convalesce after surgery or illness. The home had a distinguished board of directors, drawn from Marin and San Francisco society. Members included Elizabeth Ashe and Alice Griffith, Harriette Kittle, Henry Bothin himself, and Philip King Brown.[4]

Philip Brown and Elizabeth Ashe ran in the same social circles in San Francisco and had gotten to know each other through their mutual interest in the San Francisco Polyclinic. Ashe knew when neighborhood mothers got TB and how much they worried about taking care of their children while also trying to get well. She often sent the women to the polyclinic to learn about TB treatment while the kids stayed at the Neighborhood House, and the symbiosis between the two organizations fostered a great friendship.

We don't know how well Philip King Brown and Henry Bothin knew each other, but it's possible that Ashe suggested that Dr. Brown serve on the Bothin board. She also knew about Philip's plan to build a tuberculosis sanatorium for women. She told Bothin about the idea and about the doctor's search for a building site, and she suggested that a gift of land adjacent to Hill Farm would be ideal. Henry had lost a sister and two nephews to TB, so he was receptive to the idea. Once again he didn't hesitate. He carved out nearly forty acres from the original Hearst property for the new project in late December 1910.[5]

Bureaucratic officials in Marin County had no objection to Philip King Brown's sanatorium project. Constructing a medical facility on private land today would be close to impossible, but in the early twentieth century, the red tape was pretty faded. Locating TB hospital facilities in suburban or country locations was also not unusual. Everyone knew someone who was in a sanatorium, had been in a sanatorium, or had died because they couldn't go to a sanatorium. Sanatoria were not medical threats to their nearby communities. In fact, they were often an economic boon, and a small town like Fairfax could see more business for its grocery stores, restaurants, and nearby farms.

Institution builders need many things: partners who share their ideals, support from municipal officials, good PR, and a deep belief that the place will actually come together. These goals aren't hard to reach, but doors can't be opened without money, the sticking point that often dooms a great idea. Dr. Philip Brown already knew this thanks to the way his mother funded her hospital and nursing school. To get the money she needed, she turned to San Francisco's wealthy women—the wives of some of the city's richest and most influential businessmen. She knew that these men had political and financial power, but the women did too. It just wasn't as obvious.

Philip King Brown had his land, but what he really needed now was cash. So he took a page from his mother's book and turned to San Francisco's society women for help. Some had been his mother's friends. Others were the wives of men that he saw at clubs and social events, and he met a few because they supported the same charities. But he didn't see these women simply as their husbands' ornaments at glittering parties. He saw brains and talent and compassion, and he knew that many of the wives in his circle would jump at the chance to help other women in ways that went beyond their checkbooks. He believed this because of his personal history, and if he read the newspapers closely enough, he also knew he was part of a larger social movement.

When Philip King Brown started his TB class at the San Francisco Polyclinic, he realized that teaching women to sleep with their windows open or on an outdoor porch wasn't doing anything to halt the disease's progress. So he came up with the grander scheme to open a sanatorium. In doing so he was helping to move forward what historians call the Progressive movement, a reaction to the false-fronted prosperity of the 1890s that people like Mark Twain called the Gilded Age. Its falsity was in how few people were actually living the good life portrayed in popular magazines and in photographs on society pages.

Child labor, impure food, and quack medications had no regulatory hand to steer them from disaster. Western farmers were devastated by crop failures and by railroad freight rates they couldn't come close to affording. Immigration sparked crowding, and longtime citizens who despaired for their culture and their jobs voiced rage and fear. These issues boiled beneath the public veneer of a segment of society that today we call the 1 percent. The other 99 percent—working women among them—had few opportunities to change the conditions of their lives.

What sparked the Progressive movement was a massive increase in urban population, which went from 9.9 million to 30.1 million between 1870 and 1900. Big business boomed and created new jobs, but it also formed monopolies, leading to job losses. Concurrent with prosperity in the board room was the despair of the factory floor, where injury and sudden death were common.[6]

Progressives sought to transform the lives of individuals through legislation and through an early and revolutionary understanding that the conditions of one's life dictated a person's future, not an outmoded belief in the prison of heredity or class. The reformers saw the inequity around them and decided to use their wealth, power, and intellect to transform culture and daily life—not for themselves but for their servants, the homeless children they saw on the streets of neighborhoods not their own, and the workers who made their clothes.

Some took on the push for change late in life after pulling themselves out of poverty; others had faced down prejudice to carve careers out of whole cloth. People such as Supreme Court justice Louis Brandeis, journalist Ida B. Wells-Barnett, and Hull House founder Jane Addams used their personal platforms to agitate for reform. They were joined by men and women less prominent but who gave their time and sometimes their lives to causes of their own.

As the twentieth century opened and began to modernize, the Progressives created a wave of reform that transformed medicine, labor, law, and women's rights. Deeply confident, they brushed away as inconsequential old arguments and draconian statutes and began to make society anew.

Doing "charity" work was nothing new for women, especially the affluent. Throughout the nineteenth century, selfless assistance to the less fortunate was considered a moral obligation that suited women particularly. Living in their domestic sphere, women were natural nurturers, and caring for society as they cared for their children was considered an acceptable activity.

Many women took their activities to a new level in the years after the Civil War and to an even greater extent as the Progressive era loomed. Beyond doling out baskets of food to the hungry, they organized, funded, and administered organizations that were as complex as any business and that encompassed a vast range of social and cultural issues: the National American Woman Suffrage Association and the National Woman's Party; the Children's Bureau; the Woman's Christian Temperance Union; the National Birth Control League. They helped others in ways that did not overtly threaten masculine dominance over commerce, religion, education, journalism, and politics. By furthering these causes, women also consciously prodded the cause of moving themselves further into full participation as citizens.[7]

Women of means had many motivations for their philanthropic activities. Some felt that the family was the foundation of a stable society, and raising women up preserved the power of the home. Others saw their own wealth slip in hard times, such as the depression of 1893, and they discovered a subtle kinship with the shopgirls and clerks they had previously only considered commercial servants.

Then there was sheer personal drive. The leisure provided by wealth and household domestic help often led to crushing boredom in women whose intelligence and energy had made them desirable as potential wives but who were expected to tamp down these traits once they were married. Even moderately well-off women of the middle class found that their home duties did not satisfy their desire to contribute in some way to their neighborhood, city, or country. More than a half century before Betty Friedan defined "the problem that has no name" in *The Feminine Mystique*, Progressive-era women realized they had a problem of their own, and set out to solve it.

Tuberculosis experts like Philip King Brown and sanatorium pioneer Edward Trudeau also felt that women had a place in the fight against TB. In 1909 Trudeau addressed New York City's Colony Club, a women's private social organization. After summarizing the advancements in TB treatment, he told the crowd they were playing a vital role in the war against tuberculosis.

"Ten years ago a ladies' club would never have dreamed of devoting an afternoon to addresses on so unpleasant and hopeless a problem as tuberculosis, or organizing to aid in its control," he said. Women had formed clubs in the years after the Civil War and then joined together in the General Federation of Women's Clubs in 1890 to cooperate and try to solve America's problems. The myriad groups were diverse in their membership and goals, and they had specialized divisions dedicated to social issues. Men such as Edward Trudeau and Philip King Brown saw in these women a potential army of supporters for their work. Trudeau put it succinctly in his Colony Club address: "Help the tuberculosis dispensary, that center of effort of all educational and preventive measures of relief; help the district nurse; the sanatorium. Help the hospital for advanced cases, for humanitarian reasons."

He then told them they had a special obligation in the TB fight: "You who have had every advantage of environment and education will, I know, want to have a share in this great movement. Science and philanthropy are its moving forces, and you may well worship at their shrine."[8]

The women who heard this speech were in the same economic and social class as the ones Philip King Brown needed to tap for financial help. Like Trudeau, he believed that women, in their traditional nurturing roles, could support anti-TB efforts. But he also felt that the ones who had money and cultural influence could do more than just be surrogate mothers for society. They could fund institutions and influence thinking as doctors made progress.

San Francisco had its share of women's clubs, and Brown was glad of it, but he didn't need to make speeches to anonymous audiences to drum up support for his sanatorium. He simply picked up the telephone. Among those who answered, and who answered his call for help, were Mary Raymond, Jeannette Jordan, and Blanche Wormser.

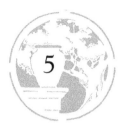

5

HERE, REST

WHEN THEIR NAMES APPEARED IN PRINT, these society ladies were called Mrs. C. B. Raymond, Mrs. James C. Jordan, and Mrs. S. I. Wormser (which made tracking down their first names a bit of a challenge). Their peers, however, knew who they were, what their husbands did for a living, how much they were worth, and where their children went to school. They were all in *The Blue Book*, the directory for everyone in society, which bore the subtitle *The Fashionable Private Address Directory*. The activities, homes, vacations, and clothing of the people in this social register were also covered in great detail in the women's pages of the *San Francisco Call* and the *Chronicle*.

But despite being hidden behind their husbands' names, these women were far from invisible. By 1911 Mary Raymond, Jeannette Jordan, and Blanche Wormser were in their forties and fifties. They were past their childbearing and child-raising years, that delightfully dangerous time when women whose ambitions had been restrained could now find full flower.

Mary Raymond was the daughter of George Perkins, the president of rubber conglomerate B. F. Goodrich, and had been born in Akron, Ohio, where the company was headquartered. Her husband, Charles Raymond, also worked for Goodrich, and they had three sons and one daughter. Sometime before 1911 they had discovered the delights of Santa Barbara and in that year bought a home called The Breakers, which Mary later renamed Westholm.[1] It was their winter place away from icy Akron, and the Raymonds soon met Philip and Helen Brown during one of their visits to nearby Miradero, which was no longer a sanitarium but the Browns' southern California family getaway. Mary and Charles Raymond had social power, in addition to money, and gave intimate dinner parties for people such as Clementine Churchill, wife of Winston Churchill, and Thomas Edison and his wife, Mina.[2]

It's easy to imagine Philip Brown finding a way to work his sanatorium idea into the conversations he had with these new friends, and Mary Raymond was soon recruited to the cause. She gave $2,000 (equal to about $50,000 today) to the doctor's building fund in early 1911.[3] And even as she and her husband commuted seasonally between Akron and Santa Barbara, Raymond kept in touch with Dr. Brown and kept abreast of his ongoing needs.

Jeannette Jordan was born Jeannette Stiles in New Brunswick, Canada, and her family was probably well-to-do, though facts are scarce. In 1892 she married James C. Jordan, a member of a very wealthy Boston family that had made its money in dry goods and real estate. The two married in Needham, Massachusetts, had a home in Boston, and had a summer place in New Brunswick. Jordan was divorced with three grown children when he and Jeannette were married, and they had no children of their own. Jordan had moved to San Francisco around 1890 and jumped into the thriving real estate market, and for a few years the couple lived in either the Palace or St. Francis Hotel. They summered in Canada but by early 1910 had a permanent home in San Francisco.

James Jordan died in August 1910 after years of being an invalid, and Jeannette went back to Boston after his death, returning to San Francisco in September. In November she gave her husband's New Brunswick home to the Canadian government to open as a tuberculosis hospital, called the Jordan Memorial Home.[4] Did Jordan waste away from TB? Was that why his memorial was a TB hospital and why the first of Jeannette Jordan's many post-widowhood donations was to a tuberculosis sanatorium? How and when she met Dr. Philip Brown is unknown, but by August 1911 she knew him well enough to give $2,500 to his building fund.[5]

Blanche Wormser, née Wertheimer, was born in Pittsburgh, and she later met and married San Franciscan Samuel I. Wormser. In 1896 he, his cousin Gustav Wormser, and Samuel Sussman established Sussman, Wormser & Co., known today as S&W Fine Foods. It was a tremendously successful wholesale fruit and vegetable company,[6] and the Wormsers lived for a time in Marin County with their son Robert before settling into the tony Presidio Terrace neighborhood in San Francisco.

Blanche Wormser and Jeannette Jordan were on Arequipa's board of managers, a group that also included Mary Holton. She was the daughter of Edward H. Miller Jr., secretary of the Central Pacific Railroad. Her husband, Luther, was in mining and electrical power, and they had a country home in Santa Barbara as well as a house in San Francisco's Pacific Heights district, where their neighbors included the Ghirardelli family, of chocolate fame. The Holtons and the Browns were good friends, and the two couples sometimes went on trips together.[7]

Isabel Dibblee was also an early supporter. She was born to the wealthy Kittle family and grew up at Sunnyside, the family property in Ross, where Elizabeth Ashe first took sickly children before she opened Hill Farm. The Harriette Kittle who gave shelter to Elizabeth's city kids was Isabel's mother.

Isabel's husband, Benjamin, was an equally prosperous Marinite who had made a name for himself as a Harvard football player before returning to California and becoming an investment banker.[8] High society in still-rural Marin was smaller but still as entwined as it was in San Francisco, and this explains how easy it was for Philip King Brown to find people willing to help him there. Bothins, Dibblees, and Kittles all wandered into one another's homes; some, such as the Dibblees, also had houses in San Francisco.

In an undated letter, probably written in 1910 or early 1911, Isabel Dibblee responded to Dr. Brown's request for money and assistance to buy furniture or linens for the sanatorium. "It will be a great pleasure to do what I can toward the furnishing of your Sanitarium and I am so glad that you called upon me for I have been greatly interested in this new enterprise. My cousins have promised to help and I only hope that we can do it all satisfactorily. It will be very easy to interest other people but I believe it better not to have too many on a purchasing Committee—We must have something a little more definite to work [with] and will you tell me when the things will be needed and first what you wish done— We will try not to be extravagant."

The letter ends playfully, and though Isabel addressed Philip King Brown as "Dear Dr. Brown," indicating perhaps that their acquaintance was not long-standing, she did have a sense of humor, which she felt comfortable enough to display: "I am soon coming to you for a prescription for taking off pounds as each week I gain a few more and am now afraid to [step] on the scales—I am afraid it is all your fault."[9]

Many of the benefactors' husbands were also supportive. This doesn't necessarily mean that the women would not have given their money to Dr. Brown without their husbands' permission. But if we look at the remarkable legacy of women's charitable work in San Francisco, it's very likely that these women had no trouble choosing to put their money, or their husbands,' wherever they wanted.

The underside to society women reaching out to the poor or the working class was condescension, whether done consciously or not. The class and cultural divide between women like Mary Raymond and a tubercular telephone operator was vast, and sometimes an offer of help was couched in language or actions that strengthened that divide. Playing the Lady Bountiful could serve the giver more than the receiver.

One example of this attitude appeared in the November 21, 1910, issue of the *San Francisco Call*, in the syndicated column called "Morning Chit-Chat," written by Ruth Cameron. Cameron was the pen name for Persis Dwight Hannah, a 1907 graduate of Tufts University in Medford, Massachusetts, who took a degree in Latin and was a founding member of the sorority Alpha Xi Delta. On the surface, the article on this November day was intended to raise awareness about the long, extra hours that shopgirls worked during the Christmas season in the major department stores. It opened with the story of one exhausted young woman who could not afford to go home and lose the few extra dollars of pay, and how the floor walker would not let her sit down, even as the hour drew close to midnight. One woman was quoted as saying she hoped she'd be dead before the next holiday.

Cameron then suggested how shoppers could help these women. "I recently heard of a sane and simple way in which one of my friends has long solved the problem of Christmas shopping," she wrote. First she suggests that women start in October, rather than waiting until December. Her friend did all her shopping before the rush season, "so she can hold herself not guilty of adding a last straw to the shopgirl's back and heart and health breaking strain."[10]

So far so good. But that is the only mention of the workers, and the balance of the article lists the other advantages of shopping early, including having the time to select thoughtful gifts and easing the burden on one's purse by spreading out gift buying over a few months. Cameron could have ended the article with a reminder that the best reason to start Christmas in October was to help overwhelmed working women, but she didn't. And here was the ever-present problem of how the giving hand could so easily be rejected by the women it was supposed to help: a benevolent motive wrapped up in high-society self-interest.

Was this how the two Marys, Blanche, Isabel, and Jeannette felt about the working-class women Dr. Brown hoped would be patients in his new sanatorium? There is no way to know, since we have few details about their other activities and even less access to their voices, because no diaries or correspondence have survived. Jeannette Jordan and Mary Holton did make the papers frequently for their other charity work, however. Jordan was a big supporter of the Columbia Park Boys Club, one of the neighborhood clubs that sprung up after the demonstrated success of the original San Francisco Boys' Club. She attended benefits and gave quite substantial financial donations to the club, which still exists today. Mary Holton's time and money went to the Little Sisters' Infant Shelter, and she served on its board for decades.

Phoebe Hearst also helped nudge the new project along. Philip King Brown was elated when he heard who had originally owned the property that Henry Bothin donated, and he couldn't wait to write to the woman he had come to call Aunt Phoebe.

"The idea of the sanitarium for the tuberculous working girls especially has taken form after my spending a year & a half looking for suitable lands. You will be surprised when I tell you that Mr. Bothin has given for this purpose some 40 acres of your old place above Fairfax. . . . Isn't it strange that part of that property should ultimately be devoted to a benevolent end."

He told her that he had enough money to pay for the building construction but not enough to furnish it.

"I am very much in hopes . . . that you may be interested in this work and perhaps feel that you want to help it develop. There will always be ways along which it can grow."[11]

Hearst worked behind the scenes during the sanatorium's planning stages and fulfilled her usual role as Philip King Brown's sounding board, although he once asked for something very specific. He wrote her another letter in July: "I am in great trouble about my little sanitarium in Fairfax. It will be ready to open about Aug 1st but it hasn't any laundry and as we are teaching that 'cleanliness is next to godliness' we are in a very bad way."[12]

Phoebe Hearst came through. And though Philip Brown sometimes used the word *sanitarium* instead of *sanatorium* in his speeches and letters, everyone knew exactly what his new venture was for.

Dr. Brown had a board of trustees as well as a board of managers, and it was made up of men and women from San Francisco and Marin County business and society. They included Frank D. Madison, of the influential law firm Pillsbury, Madison & Sutro; Henry Bothin; and William Kent, a U.S. congressman from California and a fierce early environmentalist, responsible for saving the stand of redwoods now known as Muir Woods National Monument. Philip himself was a trustee, and the group was rounded out by Harriette Kittle; Harriet Carolan, daughter of George M. Pullman, of Pullman train car fame; and

Elizabeth Ashe and Alice Griffith, the twin pillars of settlement work in San Francisco.[13]

The members of the board of managers very likely socialized together as well as managing their Arequipa duties. In 1912 they did both when they attended an unusual art event to benefit the sanatorium. That spring a painting called *The Shadow of the Cross*, by Canadian artist Henry Ault, went on display in a Sutter Street gallery. Painted in 1896, it toured a number of European galleries before arriving in San Francisco. It is a portrait of Jesus that, when displayed in semi-darkness, shows a cross looming over his shoulder. But in full light the cross does not appear, a phenomenon the artist was either unable or unwilling to explain. How the board arranged for this painting to visit San Francisco is unknown, but the gallery admission fees went to Arequipa, certainly one of the most unusual charity events ever conceived, even in San Francisco. (The painting is now at the San Francisco de Asis Mission Church near Taos, New Mexico.)[14]

Brown relied on donors and corporate officers wherever he could find them, and the men he saw in clubs and at social occasions were as important to him as the women who charged in to give him their money and their time. He chose men who had both influence and a proven track record of benevolence. However, none of them came from San Francisco's ethnic communities.

This was not a surprise to anyone. The Chinese had been reviled and shoved into a few blocks of real estate for decades. African Americans were a small population in the late nineteenth and early twentieth centuries, and while they originally saw San Francisco as a city with great potential, they were often disappointed. Labor unions and white immigrants kept them from taking the highest-paying jobs, though they still thought restricted urban life in California was better than impoverished rural life in the South.[15]

The boards that governed institutions such as Arequipa drew their members from the monied classes. Men such as Philip King Brown wanted their administrative expertise and also their fund-raising skills. Chinese and African American residents, in addition to the small population of Japanese Americans, did join and fund their own associations, but their energy and money were reserved for the unique needs of their own communities. The African American elite came from the upper reaches of the city's middle class, but they never reached the heights of white society.[16]

It was a different story for San Francisco's Jewish residents. Families such as the Wormsers were supporters of myriad charities in the city, many specifically aimed at their fellow Jews, such as the Pacific Hebrew Orphan Asylum. But their giving went beyond their coreligionists, and in this they personified a unique and little-talked-about aspect of San Francisco history. Jewish merchants and their families were among the first to make their permanent homes in San Francisco in the years before statehood. Even as the frenzy of the gold rush raged in the late 1840s and early 1850s, Jews founded synagogues, orphanages, benevolent societies, and cultural institutions as support systems for the new city they planned to call home.

While anti-Semitism did exist in San Francisco, it was much less virulent than in the cities and countries Jewish emigrants had come from. San Francisco's Jews were not restricted from any profession or place, and they were prosperous and generous, making them appealing to men like Dr. Brown. Their names appeared in *The Blue Book* and in the influential *Walker's Manual of California Securities and Directory of Directors*, a sort of social register for capitalists, published yearly beginning in 1909. Men like Henry Bothin were in the directory; he was associated with companies such as the Kilauea Sugar Plantation Co. and the Marin Water & Power Co., among many others. And so were Jacob and Sigmund Stern, the nephews of dry goods merchant and blue jeans millionaire Levi Strauss, along with many other Jewish businessmen who would donate money and goods to Arequipa in the coming years.

African American and other nonwhite residents were not listed in either *Walker's Manual* or *The Blue Book*, no matter how prosperous or influential they were. This bias was reflected in Philip King Brown's choices for Arequipa's boards as well. He was a man of his class, after all. But who knows how much more he could have done at Arequipa with the viewpoints of men and women from outside his own circle of influence.

While the board of managers oversaw day-to-day efforts, the trustees looked at the larger picture, at the sanatorium's ongoing financial health, and how the facility should change as TB treatment changed. This is consistent with how charity and philanthropy were defined in the late nineteenth and early twentieth centuries. Charity meant efforts to help individuals or specific organizations. Giving food to the poor at Christmas, or giving a donation to an orphanage, was charity. But philanthropy meant solving problems on the scale of society, changing institutions to eradicate poverty, illiteracy, disease.

The men and women who supported Dr. Brown's project with their time or money, and who made sure it stayed open, did both. Individual women left the sanatorium TB-free; this was charity, one patient at a time. When hundreds of women left the sanatorium without disease and used what they had learned there to keep themselves and their families healthy, TB lost its grip across neighborhoods and whole communities; this was philanthropy, one city at a time.

Jeannette Jordan, Mary Raymond, Blanche Wormser, and the others gave money and gifts where they saw specific needs. We can only speculate on the motivations for their involvement, but it's clear that the sanatorium was an avenue for ambition and the desire to change lives. This is how someone gets to be called a philanthropist.

Existing records show that the sanatorium's governing bodies and first benefactors were overwhelmingly female. Rarely did an institution founded by a man put so many women in charge, no matter how much money they gave him. Other San Francisco organizations with all-female boards included the Golden Gate Kindergarten Association and the Fruit and Flower Mission, which visited the sick and gave them food and, as advertised, flowers. Directors and boards of managers for groups like these were frequently made up of women only because childhood education and visiting the sick were "feminine" activities. Men generally served on the auditing committees and advisory boards. Philip King Brown himself was an advisor for the Fruit and Flower Mission. At these organizations, women ran the daily activities (much as they ran their homes) while men oversaw their financial health and gave advice in areas where they felt it was needed.

But Dr. Brown had a different idea. Although his sanatorium would treat the sick, that very female function, it was a *medical* institution, and medicine was still very much a male activity despite the growing number of women doctors opening offices in San Francisco and cities across the country. Philip King Brown's entrusting so many administrative duties to women and overseeing so many areas of the sanatorium's daily life later on shows Charlotte Brown's hand still at work.

Perhaps he also saw in Mesdames Raymond, Jordan, Dibblee, Wormser, and Holton the same impulse that had sent his mother to medical school in the first place: to move society in the right direction, to look unpleasantness in the eye instead of looking away, to feel that your life counts for something beyond your home life or your balance sheet. Involving a new generation of strong-minded women with his sanatorium honored the woman who steered Philip King Brown into his own career.

With a property deed in his hand and his bank account flourishing, Dr. Brown now needed a building plan, but he first had to decide what kind of sanatorium he wanted. The United States had hundreds of sanatoria by this time, but myriad versions of what they looked like and how they housed their patients. He may have been familiar with the most recent edition of the book *Tuberculosis Hospital and Sanatorium Construction*, written for the National Association for the Study and Prevention of Tuberculosis. It was a comprehensive guide for any individual, municipality, or organization that planned to treat TB patients, from the most ill to the most ambulatory.

Had he seen the book, he would surely have been pleased to read its description of the most favorable sanatorium site: "Every effort should be made to place patients upon sites that have natural attractions which will help to amuse and make them contented. A sloping, rolling, or hilly piece of land is more desirable than a level one."[17] Henry Bothin's gift was on the southern slope of White's Hill, the most prominent point around the village of Fairfax.

Two styles stood out among the construction possibilities. The first was a single building housing both administration and patients, with the latter cared for in wards or in a collection of small rooms housing multiple patients. The other type had one building for administration surrounded on the property by separate cottages for multiple patients. This was what Edward Trudeau and W. Jarvis Barlow's sanatoria looked like.

Philip King Brown had been corresponding with Barlow and Trudeau, and both of them gave him advice about the pros and cons of their systems. But in the end, Philip decided on the one-building-for-all program, which had advantages over the separate cottage plan. For one thing, it was cheaper to build, especially when it came to paying for plumbing, electrical power, and water. Both administrative and medical tasks could be focused in one area, and it was certainly easier on the staff to not have to traipse over a large property to go to individual cottages to see patients.

Brown told Barlow what he decided on, but Barlow tried to change his mind in a November 1910 letter: "We found that the coughing and snoring of certain patients was disturbing to others at night and each one always wants to be in one of the cottages, where he or she has a separate room to themselves. That is the reason that I felt you might have some difficulty at first in having several in one room or ward. Of course, the earlier stages you take the less trouble you will have from this source."[18]

In other words, people who have an early case of TB don't cough as much.

Next on the agenda was an architect, and Dr. Brown had many gifted men (and a few women) to choose from in San Francisco and the Bay Area. He eventually settled on John Bakewell, a Kansas native educated in Paris and at the University of California at Berkeley. He was a protégé of Bernard Maybeck, who taught at Berkeley and had helped Phoebe Hearst organize a competition to create the university's master plan in 1895. Bakewell was also a trustee of the Telegraph Hill Neighborhood Association, the umbrella organization that oversaw Elizabeth Ashe's settlement house. By 1910 he was half of the firm Bakewell & Brown, the latter being Arthur Brown Jr., one of Bakewell's fellow students at the École des Beaux-Arts in Paris. They designed homes and commercial interiors, one of which was the luxury department store City of Paris, which stood for decades in San Francisco's Union Square. They also designed the city's post-earthquake City Hall.[19]

Under Philip King Brown's guidance, Bakewell drew up plans for an efficient hospital building for the convenience of doctors, nurses, cleaning staff, and patients alike. A reporter who saw the drawings a few months later wrote about them in a *San Francisco Call* article. "The first floor will be formed of a large living and dining room, kitchens, pantries and storerooms, with a long sleeping porch for 12 patients, fitted with windows and screens. At the front of the porch will be a balcony. Upstairs will be another sleeping porch and nurses' rooms."[20]

In a regular hospital, the "sleeping porch" would be called a ward, but Bakewell and apparently the reporter knew that covering the walls nearly top to bottom with screens made the word *porch* more appropriate. Patients could put chaises on the exterior balconies to spend time in even more open air when the weather cooperated.

In his November 4 letter to Philip King Brown, Dr. Barlow wrote about screens and their value beyond just bringing fresh air into a sanatorium: "I believe you will have to have screens around your sleeping porches on account of the flies in the early morning, which all patients complain of where there are no screens." Whether Dr. Brown had already planned on screens early on is unknown, but they were certainly in place the following January.

Dr. Barlow also had some advice about flooring.

"Hardwood floors: I found these very disadvantageous because they were so expensive to keep clean and looking decently. . . . Linoleum, of course, is the cheapest to keep clean, but I believe I would paint your floors and save the expense of the hardwood."[21]

Tuberculosis Hospital and Sanatorium Construction also recommended linoleum—specifically "battleship linoleum," the toughest type available, which was used in both homes and institutions. However, in places like kitchens and bathrooms, where floors can easily get wet, tile or cement were recommended. Apparently even battleship linoleum disintegrated when exposed to too much water. For reasons of his own, or perhaps under Bakewell's guidance, Philip King Brown chose to put hardwood on the floors of the sleeping porches, though the kitchen and toilet areas did get linoleum.

Bakewell made the sanatorium beautiful as well as healthful. Architecturally his design was called "shingle" style, a motif imported from the East Coast and popularized in the Bay Area beginning in the 1890s. When it was used on homes it was known as "rustic city" style. Brown shingles helped the building blend into its surroundings, making Arequipa up to date and environmentally appropriate. Was this deliberate? We don't know, but Dr. Brown liked what he saw and was touched when Bakewell told him he would donate the plans and not charge for his work.

~

On January 12, 1911, the *San Francisco Call* ran an article titled "Phthisis Patients to Be Cared For: Modern Sanatorium to Be Built on Slope of Marin County Hill." *Phthisis* (pronounced THIGH-*sis*) was another name for tuberculosis and a surprisingly well-known word in nonmedical circles. In April the *San Francisco Chronicle* reported on the project's progress with its article "Sanatorium Will Be One of the Best Equipped in the Country."[22] It described Philip King Brown's goals for the new venture: to provide a place where San Francisco's working women and girls at risk for TB could leave the dangers of the city and let their lungs heal in country air.

This article also published the name of the new sanatorium, the first time it ever appeared in print or in public. It was to be called Arequipa.

Philip King Brown had been thinking about a name since 1910. In late September or early October of that year, he wrote to Dr. Edward Livingston Trudeau in Saranac Lake. Enclosing a copy of his "Tuberculosis Class Work" article, he told Trudeau about the plans for his sanatorium and asked if he could name it after him. Trudeau replied on October 26 with grace and modesty. He began his letter with a quick "thanks but no thanks," because apparently Brown wasn't the only one with this idea. Although Trudeau was aware of the honor, he wanted to keep the name for his own work alone. "If there are a number of Trudeau Sanitariums *confusion would soon ensue*," he wrote.[23]

Within a few months, Philip King Brown came up with Arequipa, and the meaning of the word has been a subject of speculation for decades. My grandmother Lois Downey always said that the sanatorium was named for the Peruvian town of Arequipa, a name that meant "place of rest." If that's true, why did Dr. Brown choose an obscure South American name for his California sanatorium? One popular explanation is that he was familiar with Arequipa because Harvard had built an observatory there in 1891. But he didn't study astrophysics at Harvard, and as far as anyone knows, he didn't have any friends who did.

For the most plausible story, we need to head to Santa Barbara and the Brown family home there, Miradero. Among the Browns' neighbors were Capt. Pryce Mitchell and his wife, Susan Wade, who came from a prominent local family. Mitchell had been a seafarer and spent time on both sailing and steamships.[24]

At the end of his career he worked for the Pacific Steam Navigation Company in the waters around Central America, and the first ship Mitchell ever captained for the PSNC was called the *Arequipa*. (Commercial vessels were often named for the cities in their territory.)[25] When he and Susan were married in 1899, her parents built a house for them. Wishing to give their new home a meaningful name, Mitchell decided to call it Arequipa. He told friends that the word was Quechua for "Here, rest." Whether it was or not, Philip knew the Mitchells and their home's unusual moniker, and he decided it was the perfect name for his sanatorium. At some point he decided that "Place of Rest" sounded better than "Here, rest," and this became Arequipa's official motto in the sanatorium's documents and reports, and in Dr. Brown's writings.

Resting was the last thing Philip King Brown was doing in early 1911. In addition to finding contractors to build Arequipa, and buying beds, linens, kitchen equipment, and medical supplies, he was also keeping up with his practice and his lecture schedule. He was a popular and powerful speaker, especially about tuberculosis prevention. And on March 12 he and Helen welcomed their fourth and last child, a boy named Bruce.

He also had to get the word out to potential patients. This was not a problem. They came from hospitals and from the free clinics of the Telegraph Hill Neighborhood House and the San Francisco Polyclinic. Philip Brown also talked to representatives from charitable organizations such as the Doctors' Daughters, the Hebrew Board of Relief, and the Associated Charities. He told them about the sanatorium and suggested that they note any tubercular women who came through their doors. Hannah Nolan, the factory inspector of the San Francisco Board of Health, was vigilant in the course of her work too. She helped educate the women she met and often found some who needed Arequipa's help.[26]

As autumn approached, everything was in place, including five patients who had been quietly admitted in August. And at 3:00 P.M. on Saturday, September 9, 1911, Arequipa's grand opening ceremony began.

From the day the first bed was turned down, Arequipa treated women alone. Even on the rare occasion when there were empty beds, Philip King Brown never considered filling them with men to keep the sanatorium's tiny income flowing. And patients weren't the only ones who pulled Arequipa into their lives.

The wealthy matrons who dug into their personal fortunes, the women doctors who took ferries and trains to get there just to see patients for a few hours, the nurses who lived within its walls, and the local singers and piano players who dropped in on Sundays to entertain the scared and lonely patients: all of these people contributed their personal skills and gifts to Arequipa. Though founded by a male doctor and administered later by his son, Arequipa was all about women, and it was women who kept its heart beating.

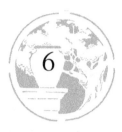

6

ART AS A TONIC

SHINING AND NEW, Arequipa had more modern conveniences than San Francisco General Hospital: sparkling plumbing fixtures, gleaming white enamel cabinets in the kitchen, the latest typewriters for the constant clerical work, telephones in the offices, and an electrical system that ensured power and light even in the worst weather. Everything in its design and contents was for the care and comfort of the patients. The doctors, however, got short shrift, because getting there was not easy.

As medical director, Philip King Brown was in charge of everything that happened at Arequipa, but he couldn't be on-site all the time. He had his own thriving practice in San Francisco in addition to his responsibilities at the sanatorium, so he needed some eyes and ears to make sure the patients were in good hands, and on a daily basis. He therefore created a rotating staff of doctors to be part of an advisory board. This group kept abreast of what was happening in the world of TB treatment and a few took turns visiting Arequipa regularly to check on the patients and their cure. All of them lived and practiced in San Francisco, which presented the physicians with a few transportation challenges.

Traveling from San Francisco to the western edge of Marin County in 1911 sounds even worse than today's traffic nightmares. First, a doctor had to make her way to the ferry terminal at the base of Market Street. There she would take a ferry across the bay to Sausalito and wait for the Northwestern Pacific electric train to take her to the Fairfax railroad station, where a staff member would pick her up in the sanatorium's horse and buggy. In 1912 a small housing subdivision named Manor was built west of Fairfax, and it soon had a railroad station just a mile or so from the sanatorium, which made travel easier. Hardier doctors sometimes walked from the train stop.

After seeing patients, consulting with nurses, and writing up notes, the doctor had to reverse the process. A half day's work at the sanatorium took up more than a day. Within a few years the sanatorium had an automobile instead of a buggy, and by the 1920s a doctor could drive her own car (if she had one) onto an auto ferry to cross the bay and then get to Arequipa under her own power. But even then, the roads out to Fairfax were still rural and still posed hazards (potholes, wildlife, infrequent gas stations) for any driver.

I use *she* deliberately here, because although Dr. Brown's advisory board had both male and female doctors on it, the ones who agreed to make the trek regularly were women. Philip King Brown found his physicians in a variety of ways. Some of them worked in or near the building where he had his own practice in San Francisco, on Hyde Street near Van Ness Avenue. He may have known others by their reputations, simply asked his colleagues for referrals, or talked to other professionals at conferences. The one thing we don't know is if he consciously chose women as the majority of his medical staff or if he chose the people who were best for the job and were willing to make the long trip out to Marin every week. Perhaps it wasn't choice at all but willingness. And it seems that the women were the ones most eager to serve.

It's also possible that Philip Brown knew that many wage-earning women had rarely, if ever, seen a doctor, and having a woman physician would ease their concerns as they tried to adjust to sanatorium life. However it happened, Dr. Brown found women uniquely suited to the work.

Many of the doctors were locals, born and trained in California, but a few were from other states and found themselves in San Francisco in time to see their careers intersect with Arequipa. These women had powered through prejudice and society's disapproval to enter the working world, though some barriers took longer to fall. In 1911, the year Arequipa opened, the San Francisco city directory still listed male and female doctors in separate categories, though they finally appeared together as "Physicians" in 1915.

Just as with his board, Dr. Brown did not hire any Asian or African American doctors for Arequipa, though there were plenty of Chinese physicians in San Francisco. Many of them were listed in the "Physicians" category of the city directory and had offices outside of Chinatown. In 1911 the directory listed three Chinese doctors and one Japanese physician. Some specialized in herbal treatments, which they advertised to white residents. Listings for 1912 included the Chinese Herb & Remedy Company, the Chinese Herb Co., and the Foo & Wing Herb Company, owned by Dr. Tom J. Chong.

Fewer African Americans took up medicine in San Francisco, however. African American men and women had few opportunities to obtain professional training for either an MD or a nursing certificate. San Francisco hospitals did not discriminate on the basis of race when it came to care, but any African American doctors who admitted patients to local hospitals were not allowed to pass through the doors to treat them. Between 1900 and 1930, no more than three black doctors or surgeons ever practiced in San Francisco.[1]

As with his boards of managers and trustees, Philip King Brown stuck with his own class, though whether this reflects his own racial views or simple convenience is impossible to know. As we will see later, however, things were very different when it came to his patients.

Visiting doctors were essential, but with Arequipa being so remote, and the possibility of medical emergencies always looming, Dr. Brown needed a resident physician, someone who would live at or near the sanatorium and be always handy. Within a few months of Arequipa's opening he found her: Dr. Hattie Bedortha, who lived a few miles away but who was always on call to tend to the patients' needs and confer with Philip King Brown during his visits.

Hattie was born Harriett Bedortha in Massachusetts around 1866. She moved to Denver, where she took a nursing degree and then her MD in 1894 at the city's Gross Medical College, later serving as an instructor there. By 1904 she was living in Los Angeles and suffering from occasional epileptic episodes, after which she took time off to rest before resuming her duties, sometimes in mental institutions. In 1906 she was living in San Francisco and was listed in a *Denver Post* article about Coloradans who went through the earthquake that April and were "reported safe."

By 1910 Dr. Bedortha was living in Napa and boarding with a family near the downtown area, possibly working at the state hospital for the insane there.[2] By early 1912 she was Arequipa's head doctor, and Philip King Brown wrote about her work in the report he would publish each year for his board, donors, and supporters. "The visits of our resident physician, Dr. Bedortha, have kept all the numerous small ailments well controlled."[3]

These ailments included everything from simple sore throats to headaches and stomach trouble. For help with more complicated issues and emergencies, especially those requiring surgery—which Arequipa was not equipped for—Dr. Brown enlisted the assistance of doctors in nearby San Rafael, who could get to the sanatorium faster than anyone coming from San Francisco and who also had privileges at Marin County hospitals.

Unfortunately, Hattie Bedortha wasn't able to stay at Arequipa very long, as her epilepsy made it impossible to keep up with an increasingly rigorous schedule and increasing number of patients. She left sometime before the fall of 1912, and her departure was a great loss to the board and the women under her care. After taking some time off, she began to work with Elizabeth Ashe at Hill Farm, seeing to the medical needs of the women and children there, which better suited her inclination and her health.[4]

Eight doctors served on the medical advisory board, though not all of them actually went out to Arequipa to check on the patients. One of them, Dr. Lewis Sayre Mace, stepped in while Philip King Brown looked for a replacement for Hattie Bedortha. He took his undergraduate degree at Stanford and then went east for medical school, graduating from New York University in 1899. He then returned to California to practice.[5] He lived in San Francisco and was on Arequipa's board from the beginning, remaining into the 1920s. He was very popular with the patients and asked some of them to write him letters about their progress. One woman named Stella went further and put a letter into verse in 1914:

> Dr. Dr. Mace; at your command
> I take my pencil in my hand
> To write my "weakly" letter.
> I'm very glad indeed to say
> I am improving every day,
> And really feel much better.

This went on for three more stanzas, ending with, "For when my 'temp.' is nearly normal / It's hard to write or feel quite formal / 'Tis so exhilarating!"[6] Philip Brown was committed to having women physicians at Arequipa, but a thoughtful and compassionate man was also acceptable.

Like other sanatorium directors, Philip King Brown gave a "Rules and Information for Patients" sheet to every woman admitted to Arequipa. It spelled out everything from payment terms to how much laundry would be done each week. Women at Arequipa were there to get cured of tuberculosis, but they were also expected to learn how to keep it from coming back once they went home. The patients were supposed to follow the rules, but not just to be tractable for the staff. They were supposed to be active learners about TB prevention, for themselves and their families, which explains the paragraph in the "Rules" sheet about not spitting on the floor.

Philip King Brown knew the women needed a distraction from their worries and that hospitals and sanatoria sometimes offered occupational therapy. But he didn't want his patients sitting in bed making useless objects just to keep their hands busy. If taking the TB cure was supposed to be a learning experience, then any other activity also needed to be practical. Dr. Brown had been thinking about this problem even as Arequipa was under construction. After investigating a variety of possibilities, he made an interesting choice: pottery.

Making pottery as therapy wasn't a new concept; he got the idea after reading about the handcraft shops that Dr. Herbert J. Hall had opened in Marblehead, Massachusetts, in 1904. Hall ran an institution called Devereux Mansion, which was a temporary home for nervous patients, much like Dr. Brown's Miradero. Pottery was one of the crafts that Devereaux offered, and not only did Hall's guests make the vases and bowls, by 1908 the venture was so successful that it was spun off as a separate commercial company called Marblehead Pottery.[7]

Handcrafted pottery had reemerged from preindustrial days during the Progressive era and was an outgrowth of the Arts and Crafts movement, which had found its way from England to the United States in the late nineteenth century. This movement was a reaction to how the machine dominated the making of household and decorative goods. Artists deplored the creative distance between the designer, the worker, and the finished product. In England, architects, writers, reformers, and designers such as John Ruskin and William Morris pushed for a return to craft and to elevating it to an art form. Morris expressed the creed for this new philosophy: "Have nothing in your homes that you do not know to be useful or believe to be beautiful."[8]

California was a crucible for the Arts and Crafts movement in America. The state's diverse natural beauty inspired architects, painters, landscape designers, and potters. The climate allowed people to enjoy the outdoors and to bring nature into everyday life. Improvements in transportation and communication meant that fine goods and new ideas could travel quickly around the United States, and both of these emerged from the Golden State, where the Arts and Crafts ideal survives still in everything from architecture to landscape design.

Pottery was particularly suited to Arts and Crafts, and American women got involved with clay work early in the movement. The Saturday Evening Girls Club was established in Boston in 1899 to help immigrant girls learn to read. In 1908 the group formed Paul Revere Pottery and began to offer clay wares for sale as a way to help newcomers make good wages in their new country. Newcomb Pottery was opened in New Orleans in 1894 under the direction of instructors at the all-female H. Sophie Newcomb Memorial College. In fact, women were pioneers in American art pottery, a field they had come to gradually after discovering the artistic and commercial delights of china painting in the 1870s. Three of America's most prominent ceramists were women: Maria Longworth Nichols, Mary Louise McLaughlin, and Adelaide Alsop Robineau. Nichols founded Rookwood Pottery Company, McLaughlin opened the Cincinnati Art Pottery Club, while Robineau was the owner and editor of the influential magazine *Keramic Studio*.[9]

After reading occasional articles in medical journals about Dr. Hall's work at Devereux Mansion, Philip King Brown decided that he could easily create a pottery works on Arequipa's grounds. The sales potential of the pieces gave him another idea: his patients could sell their wares while they were still at the sanatorium, and the money they made could help pay for their treatment. Creativity, therapy, financial means: clay craft could do as much for patients as skilled nursing and fresh air.

Pottery and tile production would be the one area in which Philip King Brown relied on men instead of women, as business managers and artistic directors or advisers. He knew many talented women were engaged in pottery work, but we don't know if he ever talked to them about bending their skills to occupational therapy at Arequipa. All the pottery directors Dr. Brown engaged were men who were either between jobs or willing to change the ones they had. Were women unable or unwilling to do the same? The ones most qualified to undertake the work he had in mind already had thriving careers or were in charge of their own pottery lines. Making that happen had not been easy, and perhaps they were unwilling to give up the autonomy of their own art and business to work for someone else.

As usual, Dr. Brown needed money to get the pottery going, and some of his most generous donors, such as Mary Holton and Mary Raymond, were tickled by the idea, so they agreed to underwrite the initial expenses. Once the money was in hand, Brown then needed equipment. He knew about the beautiful work being done in Detroit at Pewabic Pottery, under the guidance of Mary Chase Perry. He contacted her and bought a kiln, a pottery wheel, and some tools, which arrived around the beginning of October 1911.

Helen Brown wrote a history of Arequipa Pottery's early years, and she was very blunt about its beginnings: "Naturally Dr. Brown and his friends who were interested in the project were absolutely ignorant of the ways and means of pottery making."[10] So it was absolutely necessary to find a ceramist who was interested enough in Brown's scheme to move to rustic Marin County and teach tubercular women how to throw clay. And in October, just as the tools and workroom were coming together, Philip King Brown found Frederick Hürten Rhead.

Born in England in 1880, Rhead was the latest of six generation of ceramists, getting his clay education in his native country. He moved to the United States in 1902 to work with famous American artists and pottery firms, including the Roseville company of Zanesville, Ohio, whose pottery from later years lines the shelves of many a home and antiques store today. In 1909 he moved to the St. Louis suburb of University City to teach at the People's University there.

In October 1911 he was on a lecture tour in the Bay Area and heard about Arequipa. He offered to take on the job of pottery director because he wanted to stay in California and because the People's University was closing and he needed a job. The deal was quickly made; Philip King Brown agreed to give Rhead and his wife six months of living expenses in exchange for their help in starting up Arequipa Pottery. The couple moved into a cottage on the sanatorium grounds.[11]

While Dr. Brown was looking for his director and negotiating with Rhead to start up the pottery, he asked one of his friends to teach the first patients in residence how to make baskets, which was another staple of occupational therapy. Actually, Ynés Mexía de Reygadas was more than a friend. She was one of Philip's longtime patients.

Ynés Mexía was born in Georgetown, in Washington, D.C., in 1870, the daughter of Enrique Mexía, who was in the States representing the Mexican government under President Benito Juárez. Her mother was Sarah R. Wilmer, who came from a wealthy Catholic family in Baltimore. The Mexías moved to Texas when Ynés was about a year old, and when she was nine her parents divorced. Enrique moved back to Mexico, and his daughter went to Philadelphia with her mother and her six half siblings from her mother's previous marriage.

Ynés was educated in the East and in Canada, and in the late 1880s she went to Mexico to live with her father. She married a young German-Spanish merchant, who died suddenly after a few years. She then married Augustín de Reygadas, a much younger man. Ynés was emotionally unsuited for relationships though. She was a clever businesswoman and managed the Mexican ranch she owned quite well when she was between marriages. But once yoked to de Reygadas, she retreated into depression.

After she had a nervous breakdown in 1909, her doctor advised her to leave Mexico and go to the United States. He knew a very good doctor in San Francisco who could help her: Philip King Brown. Ynés and her husband moved to the city, and she began to talk to Brown about her problems. Eventually, Augustín went back to Mexico; Ynés divorced him years later.

We don't know what kind of diagnosis Philip King Brown gave Ynés, but he thought she needed to engage more with the world. In the fall of 1911 he asked her to learn the basics of basket making, take the train to Arequipa a few days a week, and teach the handiwork to his patients. As the days grew cooler and the pottery works came closer to completion, both Ynés Mexía de Reygadas and her charges found peace as they worked the reeds and willow branches into form.[12]

~

Dr. Brown made one thing very clear when he talked with people about the pottery plan. There was no danger that the TB bacillus could be transmitted to anyone who bought the finished products.

For one thing, women who worked in the pottery could not have a cough or a temperature higher than ninety-nine degrees. In other words, they couldn't be contagious. These women were in the final lap of their cure, and if their symptoms didn't come back they would soon be discharged. Also, the pieces were fired in a white-hot kiln, guaranteed to kill anything that might linger in the clay. But for the most part, Dr. Brown found that his financial backers and the owners of the San Francisco gift and department stores who agreed to sell the pottery were not worried about germs.

Once approved, a patient could put in between one and five hours per day at the pottery, but she had to build this time around a daily rest period. And patients could work only during the week, because Saturdays and Sundays were also purely for rest. Women could spend time making clay forms even if they had no intention of selling their pieces. Not everyone had artistic ability, but Dr. Brown felt that anyone who worked in the pottery would benefit from the creative activity, if only to keep their minds free from worry.

Frederick Rhead got the production end of things up and running soon after his October arrival. He found a good supply of red clay about two hundred feet from the pottery building, which will not surprise any Bay Area gardener. The rest of the clay came from deposits near Lincoln, in Placer County, California's old gold rush country. There was also help over the hill in the next valley.

Elizabeth Ashe's Hill Farm was thriving as a place of convalescence for the sick and a country retreat for weary city children. This meant that plenty of preteen and teenage boys were on hand doing chores around the property.

Dr. Brown asked Ashe if some of the boys would like to do heavy lifting work in the pottery shed and dig around the grounds for clay deposits. It is easy to imagine how much fun city boys had digging in the mud. Brown never lacked for volunteers, and the women enjoyed having the young people around.

The patients always formed and decorated the clay pieces. Rhead trained the women who qualified to work in the pottery, and by April 1912 the ones who showed the most natural skill were making pieces to order and making money. The shed they worked in was screened, mirroring the sanatorium, so that no clay dust would linger in any lungs. The women worked the wheel, carved designs into the wet clay, and applied glazes, handing their work to Rhead or the Hill Farm boys to put into the kiln.

Sometime during Rhead's tenure, the women began to carve or paint a unique mark on the bottom of the vases and bowls. No one is absolutely sure when the mark first appeared, but most scholars agree that Rhead came up with the idea. The design showed a stylized tree hanging over a large pot surrounded by the words "Arequipa California." Rhead had a fondness for trees in his own designs, which could explain the first use of the mark. The design varied on each piece because the individual patient usually drew or carved the design herself, reflecting wildly divergent skill levels. All pottery had identifying marks, and the fact that Arequipa Pottery joined these ranks means that both Rhead and Dr. Brown believed the enterprise had a future.

Brown also pressed one of his old friends into service. Bruce Porter came up with simple designs that the patients could carve into the pots and bowls, and he often came out to the site to help the women personally. His own artistic career had taken off and in an astonishing variety of media: painting, stained glass, landscape architecture. But he always found time to help his old Les Jeunes compatriot.

Porter and Brown had many mutual friends, and one of them was the Reverend Joseph Worcester, who had arrived in San Francisco in 1864 from Boston. He was a minister of the Swedenborgian Church, founded in the eighteenth century by followers of Swedish philosopher Emanuel Swedenborg. Among the church's core beliefs was the idea that the natural world was a physical manifestation of the divine. Therefore, when art of any kind reflected or respected nature, it too came close to expressing the true nature of God.

Worcester was also an aspiring architect and a devoted adherent of the principles of the Arts and Crafts movement, which he felt blended perfectly with his religious faith. He built a home across San Francisco Bay in the suburb of

Piedmont and got to know everyone in the region who was living the Arts and Crafts ideal: architects Bernard Maybeck and Julia Morgan, painter William Keith, and nature writer and early environmentalist John Muir, among many others. In 1887 Worcester moved back to San Francisco to lead the Swedenborgian congregation there, and in 1894 he began to build a new house of worship at Washington and Lyon Streets, in today's Presidio Heights neighborhood. Worcester found Bruce Porter through his artistic friends, and he helped the reverend realize his vision of a structure that would blend nature and religion. Porter drew an outline for the church building and also designed its stained-glass windows.[13]

Dr. Brown may have met Worcester through Bruce Porter, but they may also have found each other through mutual charitable interests. Worcester founded the Society for Helping Boys and began construction of the society's orphanage the month before Arequipa opened in 1911. Given Brown's early and ongoing interest in the Boys' Club, it seems likely that the two men would have met at meetings or through a personal introduction.

Worcester was old enough to be Philip Brown's father, but the two men found much in common. The minister was interested in the pottery works at Arequipa and visited regularly. Sometimes Worcester would bring boys from the orphanage out to Arequipa, and they occasionally helped dig clay around the property. Then in his late seventies, the pastor sometimes found the trip tiring, so Dr. Brown fixed up a cottage on a small rise above the pottery buildings where he could spend the night before heading back to San Francisco. It was soon dubbed Mr. Worcester's Cottage.[14] Philip had also honored his friend when his youngest child, Bruce, was born, giving him the middle name Worcester.

When he passed away in August 1913, Joseph Worcester was mourned not just by Philip King Brown but by the entire artistic and religious community. He left a sizable estate of $50,000, most of which went to nieces and nephews, but he also remembered his charities. He owned sixty acres of property farther north near Sacramento and left the land and a bequest of $5,000 to the Society for Helping Boys. He bequeathed $500 to Bruce Porter for a purpose the two men had apparently discussed in advance but that the will did not spell out.[15]

∼

As the weather warmed, patients sat outdoors to carve the wet clay on vases and bowls. When Philip King Brown visited Arequipa he sometimes brought little Phoebe with him; she was seven years old in 1912. While her father looked in on his patients, she wandered the grounds, enjoying the trees and the occasional deer sighting. She sometimes went into the pottery building, and the women helped her work the wheel and make carvings in some of their own pieces. These were the best days for the mothers who had to leave their children behind to take the cure.[16]

By the autumn of 1912, newspapers around California were taking notice of the pottery. One of the best headlines was in the *San Francisco Call*: "Wooing Life Anew at the Potter's Wheel." Reporters understood that the women were not making pottery just to have something to do. They realized the work affected the patients' health directly, whether by bringing them peace through art or by paying for their beds when it sold.

Newspaper articles never mentioned how the women felt about their time in the pottery. Visiting reporters praised the setting, the beauty of the vases, the overall concept of the pottery, and how it was supposed to work within the women's lives, but either their voices are absent or others speak for them. In one *Call* article, for example, writer Ida L. Brooks tells Frederick Rhead that if she were at the pottery, she would want to play there all day. He replies, "We do play here all day."[17]

But journalist Eloise Roorbach, who wrote articles for the magazine the *Craftsman*, truly understood the meaning of Arequipa pottery. This makes perfect sense, because the journal was edited and published by Gustav Stickley, one of the giants of the Arts and Crafts movement.

In 1913 Eloise was wandering down a San Francisco street and saw Arequipa vases for sale in a large gift store. She went into the shop to examine them more closely, as they didn't look like any of the fine china and other shiny products on the shelves. The owner told her about Arequipa, and she was so intrigued that she decided to visit a few days later. She took the ferry and the electric train to the stop at Manor, walking the rest of the way.

In her article "Making Pottery on the California Hills: Art as a Tonic," published in June, Eloise wrote about the lively, chattering women reading and sewing on the outdoor balconies. She introduced herself to Rhead and watched him and the women making the pieces she had so admired. Unfortunately, she did not mention any conversations she might have had with the women, but her article was welcome advertising for the pottery, especially being written by a woman.[18]

It is possible that some patients saw their pottery time as a diversion, even as entertainment; absent letters or diaries, we don't know how anyone really felt about this part of the TB cure. But underneath it all was the desire to produce items that were good enough to be sold, because that meant money that patients could put aside for their treatment. It may have been playtime for a professional ceramist like Rhead, but to the women who worked beside him in the pottery shed, and who hoped that someone would buy a vase or bowl, those few hours a day were deeply serious.

~

Philip King Brown needed a live-in manager or superintendent, and from 1911 to early 1912 two different women took on this position, but they only stayed a few months. An important part of the job was buying food and supplies for the sanatorium, and the unnamed women were apparently not familiar enough with purchasing or didn't know how to find local vendors. Elizabeth Ashe, who had been running Hill Farm since 1905, stepped in to take over, and a few of the female benefactors did the same. Then, on February 1, 1912, L. Nora Harnden was hired as the new superintendent, and things began to look rosier.

Nora—she always signed her name L. Nora, the *L* being for Lucy—was born in Alameda, near Oakland, in 1871. Her family was from Massachusetts but for an unknown reason had moved to the Bay Area. A brother was born in Alameda in 1877, and then the family relocated to Hawaii sometime before 1881. Two more brothers were born in the islands.

By 1906 Nora Harnden was back in California, working as a nurse in Alameda, though where she got her training is not known. She apparently worked in private homes, and how Dr. Brown found her is another lingering mystery, but by February 1912 she was living in a cottage on Arequipa's grounds and had begun her duties there.[19]

Her letters to Philip King Brown from the first few years are full of practical information and questions since, in addition to keeping up with Arequipa's food and linen needs, she managed the laborers who came to the sanatorium to work around the property and make improvements to the pottery buildings. She told him about everything that went on around her, and in July 1912 they corresponded about a serious situation with one of the patients. Dr. Brown had to jump in not only on behalf of this individual woman but in defense of the whole medical profession.

He corresponded regularly with Ynés Mexía, who was assisting Blanche Wormser at Arequipa. Blanche was the secretary to the board of managers and felt it was important to be on-site as often as possible. That summer Dr. Brown had to fire a nurse named Wheeler because she was a front for what he called a "quack doctor" operating out of Oakland. He wrote to Ynés about the situation on July 23: "She got addresses of all the girls who left and tried to get them as well as several in the sanatorium to go to this man. She was caught at it when she took Dove C. away and after she was fired she wrote to some of the girls who were under her influence and tried to make trouble."

Dove was a twenty-eight-year-old working woman from Fresno who was admitted to Arequipa sometime earlier in 1912. Philip King Brown was outraged when he heard she had been seduced away from the sanatorium by someone who advertised that he had a new type of TB cure: medicated snuff. His name was C. Hilary Young, and he was not a medical doctor, which made Philip even more concerned for Dove, who was very seriously ill. He then asked Ynés Mexía to do something a bit underhanded.

He wanted to find out exactly what the treatment was and how much it cost, so he told her to call Young's office and pretend to be inquiring about a friend. "You might even ask to see Dove," he continued in his letter.[20] Ynés somehow convinced Dove to come back to Arequipa, but Nora Harnden was shocked at her condition when she picked her up at the train station in Fairfax. She wrote to Dr. Brown immediately: "She looks like death—& inhales a powder *all* the time—I did not leave her with the girls at all but she saw & talked with them. She is killing herself as fast as she can."[21]

When Dove was told she couldn't stay at Arequipa and take the "powder," she left and never came back. Although this must have been very upsetting to the staff, her departure was described tersely in the 1912 annual report's list of discharged patients: "Dissatisfied and went to a quack in Oakland."

The following year, C. Hilary Young was hauled before the state board of medical examiners about his TB-curing snuff. The judge was actually lenient with him. "There is no evidence to show that Young ever called himself a doctor or allowed people to call him doctor, and there is testimony here to show that his preparation was helpful in several cases," he said. Young pleaded guilty to a technical violation of the law and was given three months' probation. Dr. Brown never wrote about Young again, but this verdict must have truly irritated him.[22]

~

When the sanatorium had opened in September 1911, twenty-four beds lined the wards. By October, twelve patients were taking the cure, with more coming in every week. Before the end of the year, there was a waiting list. Brown, the trustees, and the board of managers realized that they would either have to start turning patients away or build a new wing. When Mary Raymond heard about the problem, she offered to pay for the addition, which she gave in memory of her father, who had died in 1910. John Bakewell was put into service again to design an extension that would mirror the beautiful, brown-shingled building that sat so perfectly on its wooded and peaceful site, and new patients were installed by mid-1913.

Despite the increase in patients, Nora Harnden managed to keep operations in hand. And anything that even remotely affected Arequipa made its way into her letters to Dr. Brown. In the summer of 1913 a huge fire roared on the slope of Mount Tamalpais, which dominates central Marin County. Although it did not immediately threaten the sanatorium, everyone felt its effects. Harnden wrote to Brown on July 10: "The fire on the Mt. has made it dreadfully hot of course, & is driving all the wild animals down this side & the whole of the other side is burned. I saw a deer in the road yesterday and people say the snakes are plentiful."[23]

Over the next couple of years, Nora Harnden continued to report on issues with the electrical system and the water pump as necessary, and she was very enthusiastic about a visit from Jeannette Jordan, who had donated some rattan rocking chairs and new dishes. She took a vacation to Hawaii in the late spring of 1914 to visit her brother Robert, who had entered the diplomatic service. But she was rapidly becoming one of Philip King Brown's least favorite employees.

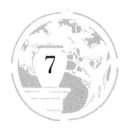

TILE AND TROUBLE

PHILIP KING BROWN THOUGHT THE WORLD of pottery director Frederick Rhead. Helen Brown, on the other hand, thought he was a disaster.

She noticed that Rhead was now spending less time helping the women make pieces they could sell and giving more attention to the few who showed artistic promise. He even brought in professional ceramists to make some of the vases and bowls, which was completely contrary to Philip Brown's vision. Stores were selling Arequipa pottery by using advertising language such as, "These artistic pieces for your home mean a livelihood and happiness to sufferers."[1] If real ceramists were making the pottery, the whole reason to buy it went away. And this took money from the purses of patients, the ones who needed it most. By May 1913 even Philip Brown could see that the pottery wasn't thriving, and after a tense meeting, Rhead agreed to resign.

By summer, thanks to the collective work of Helen Brown, her husband, and the board, Arequipa had a new director: Albert L. Solon, another Englishman with ceramists throughout his family tree. Born in 1887, he was descended from Solons who were originally from France but who took their pottery skills to England in the early nineteenth century.

Two of his brothers were already in the United States by the 1910s, and Solon joined them, ending up in southern California working as a chemist for brick and terra-cotta factories. He was making surveys of the various native clays there when he heard about the Arequipa job, very likely from Rhead. He wrote to Philip King Brown, presenting his credentials, and Brown offered him the job of pottery director starting in July.[2]

His first task was to reorganize the entire operation, and according to Helen Brown, he and Bruce Porter smashed many of the "hideous" pieces of pottery that Rhead had left behind. But Solon had better business sense than his predecessor. He built a separate room just for the glazing process, installed shelving in the kiln shed so that pieces could dry more quickly, and put a new roof over the largest kiln. It took nearly a year to straighten out the production and the physical structures, but even Helen was pleased with Solon's progress and his commitment to the patients.[3]

He may have been easier to work with too, as he had a sunny and engaging personality. He was charming and smart, and never wanted to take life too seriously. Even better, he was willing to drum up support for the pottery whenever he could. In April 1914, for example, Solon spoke to a Marin County women's club about the work being done at Arequipa and brought a few pieces of pottery with him to show off to the assembled matrons. The chairwoman of the meeting was enthusiastic about his visit and about the idea of selling pottery to benefit tubercular "girls," adding a boosterish comment of her own to convince club members to buy Arequipa wares: "Californians should help to push this industry of Californian labor with California material."[4] By the time the meeting was over, Solon had sold nearly all the pieces he had put on display.

A few months earlier, Helen Brown had rented a small office in San Francisco so that she could manage the pottery's paperwork, though she eventually turned that over to a friend who needed a job. By April 1914, gift shops in Santa Barbara, Monterey, and Oakland carried Arequipa pottery, and the magnificent St. Francis Hotel on San Francisco's Union Square ordered seventy-five flower vases for its dining room.

Arequipa also kept up with changes in its own neighborhood. The town of Fairfax was listed in Arequipa's annual reports and other paperwork as both its physical location and its mailing address until 1914. In that year, the cover of the annual report declared that Fairfax was the post office location but that the railroad and express stop was in Manor, the subdivision built in 1912 just a mile from Arequipa. This was an important distinction, because Manor was more convenient for physicians, board members, and visitors, something that was important to Dr. Brown.

San Francisco was planning a world's fair for 1915 to commemorate completion of the Panama Canal and its own resurrection from the fiery despair of 1906. It was called the Panama-Pacific International Exposition, and Arequipa's board raised the $550 entry fee so that the sanatorium could have a booth at the fair, which opened in February. The PPIE was both entertaining and educational, with exhibition palaces grouped around a central tower and long streets known as courts. Here, visitors could see a working model of the Panama Canal and models of Yellowstone National Park and the Grand Canyon, among other wonders.

Arequipa's booth was in the Palace of Education and Social Economy and featured a model of the sanatorium and a display of the pottery made by women who were still taking the cure. Former patients who had shown skill at pottery making demonstrated the process and threw clay on the wheel while rapt audiences watched. They were paid eleven dollars a week to work at the fair and could put their finished products up for sale. They also got a 10 percent bonus on anything they sold.

One of them was a young woman named Verena Ruegg. She was born in San Francisco in 1895, and her Swiss-born father was the bookkeeper for the luxury goods store S. & G. Gump (later known as Gump's). In 1913 Verena developed tuberculosis. She entered Arequipa in July and was discharged as "apparently cured" in April of the following year. Helen and Philip King Brown kept in touch with her because she had shown more natural artistic talent than many of the other women who tried their hand in the pottery. When it was time to recruit former Arequipa pottery workers to work in the PPIE booth, Verena was at the top of the list.[5]

To make sure that visitors understood the correlation between pottery and the TB cure, Dr. Brown posted a chart that compared cure rates between the women who worked in the pottery and those who didn't; the former being faster than the latter. The women who were still at Arequipa made pottery specifically to sell at the fair, and since the PPIE drew viewers from all over the country, stores in Chicago and New York soon placed orders for their shelves. Sales were good enough to cover the $150-per-month booth fee for the run of the PPIE. The pottery also won awards: two certificates of honor, two gold medals, and one bronze medal.

Under Albert Solon's management, the pottery was now making a profit. He kept up the good work through the spring of 1916 but threw the enterprise into chaos again when he told Philip King Brown that he would be leaving in May. The San Jose Normal School (now San Jose State University) had offered him a teaching position, and after three years at Arequipa he needed a change. Philip and Helen Brown were sad, but they understood, and Solon helped them begin the search for their next pottery director. With his connections, it didn't take long for Fred Wilde to take up the mantle of command.

He was born in England in 1856 and came to New York in 1885 with his family by his side and some glaze formulas in his suitcase. He worked for a number of tile companies in New York, New Jersey, and Pennsylvania and was then lured to southern California, where he worked for the company that made tiles for San Diego's Panama-California Exposition, the rival to San Francisco's PPIE. He was on-site and at work at Arequipa by September 1916.[6]

But five years into his pottery program, Philip King Brown began to notice that sales were dropping. He thought it was because tastes had turned and customers wanted the perfection of the machine in the ceramics they bought for their homes. People were less inclined to buy the products of less skilled hands, even for a good cause. But uniformity and beauty could be found in ceramic tile, which was Wilde's specialty. Wilde introduced new designs for the tile and also introduced a more precisely drawn version of the traditional tree and vase motif. (No one knows who originally drew the artwork.)

With Wilde now at the helm and the focus of the work changing, Dr. Brown had hopes that the women could start making money again. And for a while, they did.

Mary Raymond helped out by paying for the women to produce tiles for a terraced patio outside the new wing in 1916. She, Mary Holton, and Jeannette Jordan also donated money for operating expenses to keep the pottery open. In 1917 Anna Dorinda Bliss of Montecito placed a huge order for Spanish-style tiles. She was married to H. W. Bliss, an official of the St. Paul & Duluth Railroad, who was also a celebrated attorney. In 1916 they built and named their home Casa Dorinda. It's very likely that the Bliss and Brown families met on an Alaskan cruise that year. It's also possible that the Raymonds or Jeannette Jordan introduced Anna Bliss to Philip King Brown and also suggested that she fill her Spanish colonial home with handmade tiles. Anna Bliss was deeply philanthropic, and the idea that her purchase could benefit tubercular working women was very appealing.[7]

∾

Dr. Adelaide Brown, Philip's sister, was a constant female presence on the advisory board from Arequipa's beginning, and so was Dr. Emma K. Willits, who added visiting physician to her duties in 1917. She was just three months younger than Philip King Brown, born in Macedon, New York, in 1869. She took a medical degree from Northwestern University in 1897 and immediately moved to San Francisco to work at Charlotte Brown's hospital for women and children. She lost all her possessions in the fire of 1906 but pulled herself together, living with another physician and her family for a few years.

Dr. Willits was a very modern woman. In 1910 she bought an electric car at the Oakland Auto Show, but it was wrecked the following year when she was hit by a speeding car a few blocks west of downtown San Francisco. She was tossed out of her own vehicle onto the sidewalk, and her car then shot through the air, smashing a fire hydrant, which sprayed water all over her prostrate body. Two police officers helped her up and tried to convince her to go to the hospital, but she refused. She hailed a taxi and went home, and if she was injured, she apparently ignored it.

She was also very outspoken. Soon after she started her job at the children's hospital, a visiting male physician saw Dr. Willits holding a retractor. "What do you expect to do with such small hands?" he asked her. She replied, "I will use skill and not brute force."[8]

Adelaide Brown probably recommended Dr. Willits for the advisory board work at Arequipa, as Brown was still very much involved with her mother's hospital and knew the work that Dr. Willits was doing there. Taking on the job of visiting physician meant extra work on top of an already busy practice. Any physician who agreed to this kind of schedule had to be a master of the balancing act, which perfectly describes Emma Willits. She came out to Arequipa once a week and spent an entire day overseeing the work of the nurses and examining patients for signs of either improvement or decline.

Things were going swimmingly on the medical side of Arequipa's management, despite the staff departures and changes, but tensions had started to build between Nora Harnden, some of the patients, and Philip King Brown himself. Her previously chirpy letters were now dark and troubling. In August 1915 Nora Harnden wrote to Dr. Brown about her feelings:

> I have given the best of me to you & Arequipa (maybe the worst too) for three years & a half & am willing & anxious to try for six months more—If I can not by that time, I should like to leave at the end of my fourth year—or sooner if you like. In the mean time, I am willing to do anything you want me to & will gladly help any one you may find. . . . I admit a great deal is my fault but I can not take the whole blame, & think I have a great deal of excuse.[9]

Whatever the problem was seems to have settled itself, because Harnden stayed on the job and over the next two years no existing letters touch on this subject. But that changed again in August 1917. On August 20 she wrote a hasty, short note to Philip King Brown: "Do you want my attitude towards you in regards to

Arequipa entirely impersonal? I have felt the place was yours, & have kept it as personal as I could—I can change that if you so desire."[10]

Was Nora Harnden imposing her personal will and attitudes on her work instead of managing the way Philip King Brown wanted her to? Were her early years on the job a reflection of her own personality and was that no longer what Philip wanted? A poem written by a patient in December 1912 gives us a hint of Harnden's character and possibly a reason why she might have clashed with Philip or the patients and staff: "There are other attendants at the Sanatorium, whose names I have not mentioned / But leaving them out was never my intention / Chief Nurse Miss Harnden is a woman of rare ability, taste and judgment, and desiring of much praise / A strict disciplinarian, but just, kind and true / Miss Harnden, here is my thanks to you."[11]

As superintendent she was in charge of the administrative details at Arequipa and should not have been imposing discipline on either the patients or the staff. She was a trained nurse and perhaps did undertake some of those duties, as the poem says. But she was very clearly an administrator, and her name never appeared on any list of Arequipa's medical personnel. Perhaps the clash between her training and her status was the problem. Whatever it was, it escalated as the year wore on.

On November 3, 1917, she wrote again to Philip King Brown:

Your self-addressed envelope to me this morning was a terrible disappointment, for I hoped it would contain a word of encouragement to me. I cannot sleep at night & hate to be alone in the daytime, for I can not believe that you really mean what you said—that *all* the troubles at Arequipa have been entirely my fault. There has been an impossible situation which no one could know fully unless on the spot & after the love, time, energy, strength & health I have given to you & Arequipa, I could not stand it. I can not believe that my 5½ years' work has been worse than nothing, but if you really believe so, I can not go on with the work. I know my faults & am as sorry for them as you say you are for yours, but I do not believe I have been as bad as the reports which you have had from the worst trouble makers, & the girls & women with an ax to grind, have given of me.[12]

This was not the best way to approach Philip King Brown. There are hints in his correspondence with Ynés Mexía that he found emotional women difficult to deal with. Ynés had a very real problem with depression and had been suicidal in her teen years. Once she was under his care, Dr. Brown sent many letters encouraging Ynés to curb her nervous temperament. She had a duty, he said, to find and hold tight to the joys of life. This same attitude comes through in his writings about the value of occupational therapy:[13] calm emotions, as well as new vocations, were supposed to flow from any work of this kind. Illness was better managed with a peaceful mind.

It's easy to discern a little of the archaic male doctor's prejudice against "hysterical" women, and the difficulty in managing them, in Philip King Brown's character. However, he may have just been expressing himself badly, because the source of this insistence on calm emotions came from his interest in—and adherence to—the Emmanuel movement, a fairly new philosophy that wedded medicine and religion.

The Emmanuel movement began in Boston in 1906 when the pastor of the Emmanuel Episcopal Church, Elwood Worcester (no relation to San Francisco's Joseph), first held "classes" in the spiritual treatment of illness after he started counseling tuberculosis patients about the emotional toll of their disease. Worcester had graduate degrees in both psychology and philosophy and had long felt that the church should do more to minister to the sick. He consulted with a neurologist to make sure his ideas about healing were sound and then began to reach out to parishioners who needed counseling about everything from physical illness to emotional trauma. The program, which offered group therapy, individual therapy, and visits by social workers, is considered by many to be the first time alcoholism was treated as a disease rather than a moral failing.

Three years later there were Emmanuel programs all over the United States. In January 1909 the Reverend Worcester came to San Francisco to oversee the start of a special psychology clinic based on Emmanuel's principles at St. Luke's Hospital and to attend the annual meeting of the Protestant Episcopalian Church.

Philip Brown had probably heard about the movement from one of its early medical supporters, Boston native Dr. Richard Cabot. Brown and Cabot were classmates at Harvard Medical School, and they remained friends throughout their lives despite living on opposite sides of the country. Philip and Helen visited Cabot and his wife, Ella Lyman, during their honeymoon, and Cabot wrote an article about Arequipa Pottery for the influential progressive magazine the *Survey* in 1912. (Philip and Helen also honored their friend by naming their second son after him.)

Dr. Brown had probably also read the book that Worcester wrote in 1908, *Religion and Medicine: The Moral Control of Nervous Disorders*. When he heard that Worcester was coming to the city, he helped organize a conference at the St. Francis Hotel so that his fellow doctors could learn more about Worcester's program.[14]

The Emmanuel system of treatment involved quieting the mind so that a minister's or practitioner's counsel could enter both the body and psyche. In this way the "patient" contributed to his or her own healing. Dr. Brown took this idea and ran with it in his own practice and with Arequipa's patients. It's unclear if Brown was raised in any particular church, but in the Emmanuel movement he found a blend of religion and science that perhaps spoke to these aspects of his personality.

Brown believed that pottery and useful occupation created the proper mental state just as well as a pastor's soothing words. But this mental state was beneficial for everyone, not only the ill, and Brown grew irritated when one of his employees could not control his or her emotions.

Such was the case with Nora Harnden's penned tirades, and whatever the cause was, she and the doctor could not talk out the problem. This was especially difficult for Brown because he was about to leave the country. But not for pleasure.

It was war.

～

The United States entered World War I in April 1917, and both Philip and Helen Brown showed support in their own ways, although until the formal declaration of war, Philip had favored neutrality. Dr. Brown used his many speaking engagements to talk about the effects of war on health, and vice versa.

He spoke to conferences in Oregon and Arizona in October of that year about rejecting men for military service because they had TB and about ways to keep TB out of the trenches once the men got to France. He also believed nurses were essential to the health of soldiers overseas and that they should get the most up-to-date training. At meetings, in articles, and in speeches, he lobbied for women to join the nursing service and for nursing schools to make sure their students were truly ready for war work.

The conflict also showed its face at Arequipa. Brothers, sons, husbands, and friends went to France and Belgium, bringing additional worries to the patients. Some women were already worried when they were admitted, having seen what war had done to their families even before they got sick. But war also brought a new purpose to the work women could do while lying in bed.

Women's groups were already organizing charity events to benefit the women and children of Europe, especially Belgium. They usually couched their events as fund-raisers for "Belgian babies," the most vulnerable victims of "Hun" atrocities overseas. During the fall of 1917 the Red Cross put on a number of these get-togethers, and women collected needed clothing for the troops and money for relief efforts.

A big auction of handmade needlework was in the works for November 1917, and Philip King Brown asked the patients at Arequipa to contribute pieces of their own. He had no qualms about asking the women to join him in this form of practical patriotism because he knew the activity would serve another purpose. Idle in their beds, the women could not do anything else to help the war effort, which could be another source of that emotional stress he knew was detrimental to a TB cure. But to make an item for sale that could save the life of a helpless child was something all the women could support, no matter what their feelings were about the war itself.

And in case anyone was worried about Arequipa's handiwork spreading contagion, Dr. Brown had the women make only items that could be boiled. In this case, they were washcloths, nine dozen of which, duly sterilized, were sent to the Red Cross in France. The auctioned needlework brought in a tidy sum for the Commission for Relief in Belgium.

The society women of San Francisco and the greater Bay Area also raised money for Belgian relief efforts. In May 1916 they organized an event called the Belgian Market, held in downtown Oakland. Women turned out in vast numbers even though it was a cold and rainy day, which the *Oakland Tribune* marked in a headline: "Society Leaders Endure Cold with Public Patrons." The women sold food, fruit, flowers, and much-welcome coffee and sandwiches. Helen Brown managed a booth selling Arequipa pottery to the shivering hordes, along with other women who offered different ceramic products for sale.

San Francisco's women held another Belgian Market in November and chose the Civic Auditorium near City Hall as their indoor venue, which kept both vendors and customers out of the fall rains. Helen sold the pottery again, and Arequipa was mentioned specifically in a number of newspapers. "The pottery that Mrs. Philip King Brown offered for sale attracted much attention and I doubt not netted a neat little fund. These lovely things are made near San Rafael, where Dr. Philip King Brown has established a sanitarium. Here the convalescents develop taste and skill and add a mite to their maintenance."[15]

Helen Brown's charity work during World War I grew from a religious faith that she had adopted as a young woman. In the mid-1890s Phoebe Hearst had started following the teachings of Abdul Baha, a follower of the Bahá'i religion (and the son of its founder). The doctrine stressed peace, religious unity, education, and equality of the sexes, which appealed to Phoebe's protégé Helen Hillyer. Helen had been reading philosophy with another deep-thinking friend, Ella Goodall, and they both embraced the faith. Helen was a seasoned international traveler, thanks to her years trailing Phoebe Hearst around the world. In 1899 she, Ella, and a dozen other American followers went to the city of Akka, now the Israeli city of Acre, where Bahá'i founder Mirza Husayn-'Ali Nuri had once been imprisoned.[16]

Helen's beliefs were the foundation for her character and her charitable work, which included women's suffrage. In 1911 she and other activists put on a variety of fund-raising events to pay for activities aimed at passing California's suffrage amendment in October. In September, as Philip was readying Arequipa for its opening on the ninth, Helen was organizing a suffrage gathering at Union Square's St. Francis Hotel.

Helen supported efforts aimed at protecting the innocent and working toward peace, even before America's entry into the war, meeting with people interested in internationalism and world peace. In December 1915 she helped bring Belgian politician Henri La Fontaine to San Francisco. He was one of the strongest voices against war in Europe and had won the Nobel Peace Prize in 1913.[17]

Bahá'i informed Helen's work with people and organizations that wanted equality and an end to war, as well as the ways she supported her husband's work. Philip's embrace of the Emmanuel movement helped him harness the power of the mind to affect the health of the body. These were both unique expressions of spiritual faith, but they added up to one very strong partnership.

Philip Brown wasn't just paying lip service to the men and women who interrupted their lives to serve their country. Although at age forty-nine he was too old to enlist, he applied for a passport in June 1918 to do Red Cross work in Europe, and he left for France at the end of the month. In France he ran into Elizabeth Ashe, who was running the Children's Bureau for the Red Cross.

Brown spent most of his time as assistant director of the U.S. Department of Medical Research and Intelligence, which supplied fields, camps, and hospitals with medical books and journals and kept doctors informed about new developments in war surgery. This was something already dear to his heart. Philip King Brown always kept up with advancements in medicine, and he thought other doctors should too.

While he was gone, his place was ably served by the sanatorium's visiting staff physician, Dr. Mary Jones Mentzer. A Pennsylvania native, Mary Jones was born in 1878 and decided early in life to become a physician, graduating from Dr. Charlotte Brown's alma mater, the Women's Medical College of Pennsylvania, in 1905. She found a man sympathetic to her career aims in attorney Edwin Mentzer, and they married in 1907. By 1912 they were living in San Francisco, and Dr. Mentzer was soon hired by Pacific Telephone and Telegraph as welfare supervisor. This meant she was the doctor for the "hello girls," responsible for the health of the telephone operators. Dr. Mentzer had a particular interest in tuberculosis and no doubt saw plenty of cases in her work at PT&T. Philip King Brown brought her on staff in 1917, but when his departure date was set, he and the board asked Dr. Mentzer to take on the medical director's duties in addition to her own. She served devotedly with skill, sympathy, and understanding.[18]

Philip King Brown was active and vocal during his time in France. He was proud of the work he was doing with the Department of Medical Research, though he was impatient with lectures and books that wasted his time and didn't add to his knowledge or anyone else's.

On October 18, 1918, he wrote a letter to the editor of the *California State Journal of Medicine* about a lecture on shock he had attended at the Biological Society of Paris. He was very clear about his opinion of the speaker, who, he said, had presented nothing new: "When a man ceases to be interesting in his discussion everyone begins a whispered conversation with his neighbor while the poor devil speaking keeps on till he has presented all of his carefully prepared notes."

He also had some exciting local news. A former pathologist from San Francisco's St. Francis Hospital had been doing work on wound bacteriology and healing, and was teaching courses on the topic at a laboratory in Dijon. Brown concluded: "We have reason to be proud too of the work done in the field and hospitals and in the Red Cross by all our California men and women. One meets them everywhere and the record of their work will bear favorable comparison to the highest standards in every field they are in. It would be hard to mention all the names and it isn't necessary. The whole story will be told soon."[19]

As busy as he was with his war work, Dr. Brown kept up with activities at Arequipa, and this included exchanging letters with Ynés Mexía about Nora

Harnden. "Did she go off on a vacation this year? I hope some end will come to the disquiet of her nervous outbreaks,"[20] he wrote on October 18, 1918. He concluded his letter by asking Mexía to hold things together at Arequipa, saying, "Do not disappoint me." However, this stern letter didn't arrive at Arequipa until well into November, perhaps even close to Armistice Day, November 11. Philip King Brown needn't have worried. Nora Harnden had left Arequipa even as he inquired about her.

She decided to travel after her unpleasant departure and applied for a passport in December, boarding a ship for Europe soon after. A woman named Mrs. Humphrey, who was described as the "house mother," took on the superintendent duties from the end of 1918 well into 1919. And the search was on for the woman who could match Nora Harnden in skill but not in character.

∽

Dr. Brown returned to California in February 1919. He barely had enough time to readjust to his peacetime life when he and Helen were flattened by sorrow.

Phoebe Hearst had been living in New York and had contracted influenza during the winter months. Her strength was slowly returning, so she came back to California to recuperate fully at her estate in Pleasanton, east of San Francisco. But the strain of travel caused her health to crumble, and she died on April 13, 1919. Multiple funerals honored her memory, and it is not hard to imagine the pall of sadness that hung over the Brown family. To Philip and Helen Brown especially, Phoebe Hearst *was* family, beyond all of the other roles she had played in their lives.

Dr. Brown also had to face the end of something else very close to his heart: the pottery.

It had creaked along when he was in France, but the wartime cost of raw materials and slowing sales made Fred Wilde see the writing in the clay. He left Arequipa in November 1918, but he arranged for a few artistic former patients to go to Arequipa and help women who were still interested in making vases and bowls. Dr. Brown came home to a much quieter pottery works, but Bay Area stores still bought a few pieces to sell to interested customers. In June 1919, members of the California Botanical Society paid a visit, and in 1921 the graduating class of a local school gave a piece of the pottery as a gift to their library. But that is the last known mention of Arequipa wares, and by early 1922 Philip King Brown had closed the clay works for good.[21]

Dr. Brown never wrote about the effect that Arequipa pottery had on the people who bought it and put the pieces in their homes. To him, the point was to create a productive, healing activity for his patients with the possibility of either financial gain or even a new career. But reporters and journalists did understand that buying Arequipa pottery was an act of compassion, even when it was cloaked in the language of art or commerce.

During the Panama-Pacific International Exposition, a writer for the *San Anselmo Herald*, from the town next door to Fairfax, heard a few women exclaiming as they looked at the pieces on display. According to the reporter, "Many ladies were surprised at the many beautiful vases—no two alike, that are on sale here and for such a good cause, the cure of tuberculosis in working girls. The work is indeed fine art."[22]

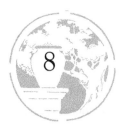

LIFE IN A LUNG RESORT

SHUTTING THE POTTERY SHED did not mean that Philip King Brown gave up on occupational therapy, or even vocational therapy, which is what he considered the pottery work to be. He studied the literature of institutional handiwork, looked at the value pottery had brought to his patients, and decided to offer other useful activities to patients who wanted something to do with their hands. As with clay, these had to be engrossing enough to keep the women interested but not strenuous enough to compromise the rest they were supposed to be getting. He gravitated toward skills that he felt the women already had and that would appeal to "the feminine instincts of personal adornment and homebuilding."[1]

Soon women who weren't already competent seamstresses could take hat- and dressmaking classes. He also revived basket making with the help of Ynés Mexía and a local man named Nicholas M. Kurtz. Originally from Germany, Kurtz was a retired rattan-ware manufacturer whose background brought a new professionalism to the art of woven basketry.[2] Knitting and crochet work were also acceptable ways for the women to spend their time. And Philip King Brown maintained his prejudice against useless busy work, preferring that women make useful items instead of "gimcracks." A few artistic patients turned to painting cards, lamp shades, and photographs, which sometimes turned into paying work after they left Arequipa.

Arequipa also did its bit for the returning doughboys. In the spring of 1918, before he left for France, Dr. Brown got in touch with Mary Patterson, head of the Department of Household Art at the University of California–Berkeley, about a partnership between the university and the sanatorium. Three students being trained as military hospital "reconstruction aides"—Elizabeth Talbot, Violet Osborn, and Eleanor Van Loben Sels—soon began a three-month stint at Arequipa to practice their new vocation.

The word we use for this work today is *rehabilitation*, and the goal was the same: to heal both the physical and emotional wounds of war and put soldiers on the road to rebuilding their lives. Occupational therapy was one of the pillars of this work, and the veterans' needs were the same as those of TB patients. Lying in their hospital beds, the men became discouraged and lost all ambition and sense of purpose. The occupational therapy director at Walter Reed Hospital, Bird T. Baldwin, said, "There is no factor that exerts more influence on a soldier in convalescence than his mental attitude."[3]

Philip King Brown agreed. Reconstruction work was another way that patients could be involved in the war effort. Orthopedists and other doctors realized the value of occupational therapy for veterans and also felt that women were especially suited to bridging arts and crafts with the military.

The three university women in training came to Arequipa once a week and taught handcrafts: beadwork, cord work, weaving, making doilies. The patients welcomed the activity because they knew that by helping the young instructors learn their trade, they were indirectly helping soldiers.

Anyone who wanted to work with the student teachers had to get a "work permit" from Philip King Brown, and it soon became a badge of honor in the wards. Within a short time the permit was dubbed a "union card" and anyone who didn't get one was slandered with the nickname "IWW." This was a reference to the Industrial Workers of the World, a union formed in 1905 in opposition to the capitalist-friendly platform of the American Federation of Labor and dedicated to advancing the rights of unskilled workers. The IWW welcomed immigrants, women, and minorities, which was a terrifying prospect to a world newly worried about socialism and communism. Using the label "IWW" as a goad or a punishment tells us everything we need to know about the political leanings of some of Arequipa's working women—and the attitude toward taking responsibility for their own cure.[4]

Many patients seemed as eager for vocational education as Philip King Brown hoped they would be. He also arranged for instructors to teach typing and shorthand and, surprisingly, to train patients to be laboratory technicians. At least three former patients learned lab technology at Arequipa and went on to good-paying jobs in the early 1920s. Dr. Brown, ever the teacher, was especially proud of how Arequipa benefited the women as a whole and did more than just heal their lungs. "Work is contagious and the creative instinct is strong in most people," he wrote. "We may not be able to make show exhibits in terms of beadwork and trinkets, but we have bigger assets in human and economic usefulness."[5]

One of Philip King Brown's success stories was the post-Arequipa life of Verena Ruegg, the former patient who demonstrated pottery making at the 1915 Panama-Pacific International Exposition. After the fair closed, Verena spent time in Boston and was listed as a ceramic worker in the April 1918 directory of the Arts and Crafts Society there. This may have just been a sideline, because by 1920 she was back in San Francisco. By mid-decade she had moved to Los Angeles and was working as a nurse, but she also studied at the Chouinard Art Institute, now the California Institute of the Arts, and the Otis Art Institute. She may have had a way with clay, but her real artistic talent was in illustration. She entered her work in exhibitions and competitions all over California. She particularly loved to draw ballet dancers and regularly visited dance studios to watch how the students moved.

She stayed in Los Angeles and in 1926 married Fred Robinson, an actor's agent, though she kept her maiden name, and soon after her marriage she seems to have turned exclusively to her art. In 1939 the Robinsons' home was destroyed by fire, though Fred managed to save most of Verena's paintings. In January 1940 her husband was killed in a car accident. As Dr. Brown taught her and she already knew, art could heal, but with her husband gone, she also had to go back to work.

By March 1940 Verena was working for Walt Disney Studios in the Promotion Department, but her talent soon got her a new position in the Ink and Paint Division. Her job was to trace the animators' pencil drawings onto cels, or sheets of clear celluloid. She stayed with Disney until February 1942, but she must have picked up the animation bug because she next went to work as a tracer for the Leon Schlesinger Studio.

Schlesinger was most famous for introducing the world to Bugs Bunny, Daffy Duck, and the rest of the Looney Tunes gang. After a few months, Verena got a new job, which was reported in the Hollywood magazine *Variety* under the headline "Lady Lenser": "For the first time in Hollywood history a gal becomes a cameraman (or camerawoman) at the Leon Schlesinger cartoon plant, where Verena Ruegg, who has worked up from a tracer's job, is lensing animations with full permission of the IATSE [International Alliance of Theatrical Stage Employees]. Shortage of manpower, due to the war, is causing a general advance of femmes in all phases of the camera art."

While there is some disagreement about who actually was the first woman to handle a camera for an animation studio, it is clear that Ruegg was early on the scene, though the job probably went back to a man when the war was over.

She continued to produce lithographs, sketches, and etchings until at least 1970. She died in Los Angeles in 1973 at the age of seventy-seven.[6]

It's doubtful that Ruegg kept in touch with Philip King Brown after she moved to Los Angeles and launched her multifaceted career. It's also likely that she was one of the few women who went on to work in the arts after her time at Arequipa. Perhaps Ruegg's time in the pottery influenced the choices she made later in life. If it did, Dr. Brown would have felt that his efforts, and the headaches the pottery works sometimes caused, were very much worth it.

Besides the doctors, the most ever-present continuity at Arequipa was the nurses. Of all the staff who served at Arequipa, they are the most elusive and anonymous. This is strange, because Philip King Brown valued nurses and their work more than the average male doctor of the early twentieth century, but they rarely if ever make an appearance in Arequipa's annual reports and are not called out by name in the lectures he gave and the articles he wrote. Despite this oversight, he had real respect and regard for nurses, an attitude that had the same source as his unusual concern for women's health: his mother.

Dr. Charlotte Brown opened a training school for nurses in San Francisco in 1880 as an adjunct to her hospital for women and children, where female doctors got vital on-the-job training. Adelaide and Philip Brown were twelve and eleven years old then, and no doubt stories about Charlotte's efforts to train women as nurses were included in many a family conversation. A few special young women likely graced the dinner table now and then as well. By the time the two children were doctors themselves, the training school was one of the most respected in the country.

Charlotte Brown thought nurses needed formal training because despite their value in homes and hospitals, many people considered them little more than servants. Opening a school was her way of making sure women were properly educated. Nursing was also another avenue for financial and emotional independence in a world still wary of the term *working woman*. She suggested that after a career nursing the sick, mature women of forty-five or older could spend their less active years teaching or serving as administrators. Dr. Brown also regularly talked to young women about saving their money for retirement.[7]

She agreed with Ann Preston, dean of the Woman's Medical College of Pennsylvania, that nurses should be considered "trained medical practitioners." Women studying nursing at the WMCP took the same classes as those studying to be doctors and also took additional classes designed just for them.

Despite some backward attitudes, women found little cultural resistance to their desire to become nurses, because the impulse to join the profession was seen as the natural outgrowth of women's ingrained inclination as nurturers. Not all male doctors agreed though, and it was only the "thinking physicians" (to quote Florence Nightingale) who realized the importance of nursing schools and the women who walked from their halls into hospital wards and examining rooms.

Nursing knowledge ran in a parallel track to medicine and was allied to that natural motherly role. Women knew the value of fresh air and proper ventilation, good food, and warmth when appropriate, and the importance of spotless hygiene. But a trained nurse had to be able to act independently in an emergency or when a doctor wasn't available. She had to recognize the meaning of changes in a patient's condition and act on them with intelligence and dispatch.

More open-minded doctors believed that nursing should be scientific. That is, anyone who wanted to be a nurse should understand anatomy, bacteriology, and physiology in order to use their reason on the job instead of simply spouting rote learning. If a nurse was lucky enough to work with this kind of doctor, she had a chance to break free of old-fashioned attitudes that saw her as a mere worker bee, eternally subservient to the (male) physician.[8]

The profession had a few specialties, and one of them was the tuberculosis nurse. In 1908 Dr. Theodore B. Sachs, head of the Sanatorium Department of the Chicago Tuberculosis Institute, had this to say on the subject: "The trained tuberculosis nurse, in her relation to physician and patient, has a much greater sphere of activity, than in any other branch of medical work. In no other case is she as equal a partner of the medical man as in supervising the treatment of a tuberculous patient, as without her the application of a proper method of treatment is frequently impossible and the services of the physician are almost useless."

Most TB nurses worked in private homes or joined a municipal visiting nurse service, which sent nurses into houses and apartments in cities and rural hamlets to check on the health and welfare of people too poor or ill to seek treatment elsewhere. Some went into the homes of former sanatorium patients to make sure they were following doctors' instructions about proper living, to keep a TB relapse at bay. As Dr. Sachs put it, the nurse "should and will be the torchbearer of light and the advocate of justice to the neglected consumptive."[9]

Nurses faced hazards against which even the most diligent sanitary measures were sometimes useless, and getting tuberculosis was one of them. Spending time in close quarters with patients made them vulnerable to TB, even more than doctors, because nurses spent more time, and more intimate time, with the sick. But there was a silver lining: nurses who were healthy former consumptives were highly prized as TB nurses. Among the many anonymous nurses who worked at Arequipa, at least two were former TB patients; they joined the staff soon after the sanatorium opened. Private nursing paid well, but it could be intermittent. Sanatorium work brought in a smaller salary, but room and board were often covered. And the work was steady, which was very appealing to many women, especially if they were self-supporting.

A few months after returning from France, Philip King Brown found a replacement for Nora Harnden. He and his board again chose a woman with nurse's training, which does make sense. An administrator with medical knowledge and experience could be counted on to understand the needs of the patients better than someone who was only a food buyer and bookkeeper. And even though Nora Harnden's nursing background had not made her immune to the potential for personality clashes, the board—and Philip King Brown too—felt that a nurse would still make the best superintendent. Ethel Steeves was hired for the job, and her tenure was much less turbulent.

Steeves was born in Canada in 1878, and her family moved to California ten years later. She entered Dr. Charlotte Brown's training school for nurses and graduated in 1901, working at the hospital for women and children while commuting there from Berkeley, where she lived with her parents. She then relocated to San Francisco and lodged with another family to be near the hospital, and that's where Philip King Brown found her and offered her the position at Arequipa. His mother's hospital and nursing school had proved to be fertile ground for finding the right woman for the job.[10]

Arequipa, or any sanatorium, needed someone at the helm who could impose order without undue emotion, because a sanatorium was both a physical structure and a concept. It was a place where doctors tried to turn disease into cure with iron discipline, but it was also a special society in which people were thrown together for the same purpose but who got there in individual ways. Within the doctor's rigid rules flowed the patients' little rebellions, a paradox of the communal life. Even while fighting off death, patients chafed at being told how to do it. Rule following and molding oneself to an artificial routine was a challenge for any patient, no matter how much she wanted to get well. A sanatorium stay was a test of will as much as a time of healing.

Everyone who had a bed at Arequipa had to learn and adhere to the ironclad daily rituals of the TB cure. Philip King Brown knew how other sanatoria operated, and he either adopted or adapted what he wanted to put in place at Arequipa. Every woman met the immovable wall of the sanatorium routine in her own way, and those who stayed found a way to cope as they found their way home.

But some patients could never adjust to being in an institution, even if it meant curing TB, and left Arequipa on their own, as patients did at all sanatoria. And except for the modernization of medical equipment and changes in doctors' attitudes toward contagion, a woman's experience of sanatorium life was remarkably similar whether she was admitted to Arequipa in 1911 or, as we will see later in the case of Lois Downey, 1927.

The discipline started at bedside. The beds themselves weren't too uncomfortable and had good, sturdy linens, though patients could bring blankets from home. (These were first fumigated.) Each patient had a table by her bed with a small bag hung from a hook within arm's reach. This was for disposing of the "paper handkerchiefs" (Kleenex before that named existed) and wax cups into which patients spit out the sputum they coughed up. These materials were taken away and burned. Patients were not supposed to carry around any tissues they had coughed into. And anyone who spit on the floor was told to leave.

Morning routines began between 6:00 and 7:00 A.M. Even the women with more advanced TB were allowed to get up, use the bathroom, and wash their faces. They took baths in a huge four-legged tub, and these were regularly scheduled and well-supervised. Then it was time for the nurses to take temperatures. One way doctors monitored a woman's health was to regularly check for fever. Any rise in body temperature, even a small one, meant that a patient still had active TB. Her body was trying to kill the bacilli, as it would any other infection. The nurse wrote the results down on each woman's chart, which by the end of the day looked like a collection of mathematical equations because temperatures were taken four or more times between breakfast and bedtime.

Patients were not passive about this part of the routine. A fever-free morning meant hope, and a two-degree rise in the afternoon meant the opposite, even though it was common for anyone with active TB, however slight, to get low-grade fevers later in the day. Medical explanations for varying temperatures didn't matter. The women wanted weeks of cool foreheads, because that meant progress.

After baths and temps, it was time for breakfast, the first enormous meal of the day. Weight loss was a TB warning sign, so building up the body and putting weight back on was a basic tenet of the rest cure. Patients were expected to send cleaned plates back to the kitchen. Unless a patient took a turn for the worse and lost ground in her cure, most women started gaining weight quickly once they entered Arequipa. Bed patients took their meals in the wards, but women who were near the end of their cure and were symptom-free could eat in the elegant, wood-paneled dining room. But everyone ate the same food.

Doctors believed that a balanced diet of proteins, dairy products, fruits, and vegetables was essential to building up a TB patient's strength. Malnourishment was one of the gateways for the bacillus in the first place. The body of a well-fed patient was better equipped to heal itself from within and build up scar tissue in the lungs, making her no longer contagious. From there, free of active bacilli and no longer feverish, a woman was well on her way to going home. Weight gain was always a good sign that the rest cure was working, though the larger number on the scale was often a shock as women realized they could no longer fit into any clothes in their closets back home.

Breakfast was generally eggs and toast, and the nurses also handed out a mandatory glass of milk for the patients to either enjoy or choke down at mid-morning. A luncheon sandwich was usually accompanied by spinach, though many doctors felt it really didn't have the kind of nutritional value everyone thought it did. But that didn't change what came out on the trays. And there was always coffee, hot chocolate, or tea to drink. The cook had Sunday afternoons off, so the patients usually had a sandwich for dinner that day. They had some kind of meat for dinner the rest of the week, either a roast or something boiled.

Nourishing it may have been, but patients never tired of remarking how much they disliked the food. Most medical directors expected the grumbling, and articles about food and proper nutrition appeared regularly in journals dedicated to TB treatment. Doctors knew they had to find a balance between nourishment and appeal, because loss of appetite can be a symptom of active tuberculosis.

Sister Rose Genevieve, one of the Sisters of Charity, who managed the Glockner Sanatorium in Colorado Springs, wrote an article for *Journal of the Outdoor Life* called "Diet in Tuberculosis." She understood the importance of food in the battle against TB and wrote with scientific dispassion about the value of milk, eggs, and vegetables, in addition to roasted and broiled meats, which she said were superior to the fried versions. Her article ended with a collection of sample menus used at Glockner, which had much heartier fare than was usually seen at Arequipa. The midday meal was the heaviest, typically something like split pea soup with saltines, baked lake trout, steamed potatoes, baked tomato, hearts of celery and pickled onions, bread, butter, and a chocolate sundae. Sister Rose felt it was the duty of the sanatorium to offer meals that were "carefully thought out, scrupulously cooked and daintily served in order to stimulate the patient's appetite."[11]

Dr. Harry Lee Barnes, on the other hand, thought that TB patients should just put up and shut up when it came to food. He was the superintendent of the Rhode Island State Sanatorium in Wallum Lake, and he published an article in *Journal of the Outdoor Life* called "Food Complaints in Sanatoria." He acknowledged that some sanatorium managers did not pay enough attention to making food palatable, but he felt that for the most part, patients were just ungrateful. He compiled a list of typical reasons for complaints about meals, which included individual likes and dislikes, ignorance, racial peculiarities concerning food and cooking, the natural tendency toward grumbling and ingratitude, a false excuse for leaving, snobbery, and fussiness. In the latter category were examples such as "one woman has complained that the pop-overs were hollow!"

But despite his belief that most TB patients were crabby, Dr. Barnes did understand why. When people who have led busy lives are forced by illness to slow down and focus on just getting well, trivial things become monumental. He concluded with a core belief shared by nearly all TB doctors, Philip King Brown included: if patients would enter into the cooperative spirit of the sanatorium, it would make it easier for their fellows, for the staff, and "to live in peace of mind, which sometimes aids recovery."[12]

Because Arequipa was in the Bay Area and near California's rich agricultural and dairy regions, Philip King Brown didn't have any trouble finding sources for nourishing food for his patients. But when he was away in France during World War I, his advisory board had to take a few steps to ensure that the women were getting what they needed. Although the Great War saw far less rationing than the one that followed, Americans voluntarily restricted their diets so that the bulk of the country's food could go overseas to nourish the doughboys now fighting there.

The board, no less than Philip King Brown, was a patriotic body, but its first priority was the health of Arequipa's patients. So in the winter of 1918 they wrote to Professor Agnes Fay Morgan, head of the Department of Household Economics at the University of California–Berkeley. They asked her to send a dietitian to the sanatorium to evaluate its menus and make recommendations for improvements that didn't violate the spirit of the war effort. Morgan sent two.

Alice Heinz and Mary Hall spent several days at Arequipa reviewing a year's worth of meal planning and then prepared a report about their findings. The board was pleased to read the sentence that summed up their conclusions: "The [diet] at Arequipa was, on the whole, so good that there was very little left to suggest."[13] Heinz and Hall did, however, say that the menus were a bit monotonous and suggested ways that frequently served foods could be prepared in a variety of ways.

Prices for fresh vegetables and fruit went up in the war years, making it difficult to keep daily costs down at Arequipa. But here again the board went into high gear. It formed a Fruit Committee, which paid the extra costs so that patients could have nourishing apples and strawberries to eat. And when the people of nearby Fairfax heard about Arequipa's plight, they regularly sent over both fruits and vegetables from their own gardens to help out.

Dr. Adelaide Brown, Philip's sister, also did her part for the patients. She had a very particular interest within the growing field of public health: the safety of the city's milk supply. In 1894, with seed money from San Francisco mayor Adolph Sutro, she had created the Milk Laboratory, where cow's milk was examined and treated so that it was free of contagion and had the chemical consistency of mother's milk (cleanliness and palatability being equally important). She was not in favor of pasteurizing milk, because at the time, the process did not remove contaminants such as the tubercle bacillus, which could be passed to whoever drank it. Her work was especially crucial in the months after the 1906 earthquake and fire. She also led initiatives to make sure that all of San Francisco's schools, hospitals, and settlement houses had clean milk to serve to the needy at their tables.

By 1919 Dr. Adelaide Brown was a member of the California Board of Health and president of the San Francisco County Medical Milk Commission. With milk such an important part of a tubercular patient's diet, Arequipa's board members asked Adelaide to examine what was being served to the residents and staff. They were relieved to learn that their milk supply was in first-class condition. Adelaide not only looked at what was delivered to the kitchen but also inspected the dairies where the milk came from and wrote a report about the best way to handle it to ensure cleanliness. The board put one suggestion into place right away: Jeannette Jordan paid for a new cement milk house.[14]

After the war was over, prices came down and cutting back was less urgent, even though the United States was still helping to provide food to the people of France and Belgium. Grumbling about food was no longer anti-American, and some of the less thoughtful women continued their ongoing campaign to comment on the daily fare, ruining a few appetites along the way.

Another pillar of a sanatorium stay was the daily rest hour. Patients at every sanatorium, from Arequipa to the Adirondacks, took a long nap every day, though the times varied. At Arequipa the rest hour was 1:15 to 2:45 on weekdays and 10:30 to noon on Sundays. During the sacrosanct rest period, the women could not get out of bed or talk to each other. Reading was allowed but not really encouraged.

A sanatorium stay was called the "rest cure" because the less movement a woman made, the more her lungs could restore and build up those all-important macrophages around the bacilli, working slowly toward arresting the active disease. For women who were used to running households, running after children, or holding down jobs, lying in bed doing nothing was either a luxury or torture, depending on your point of view and how badly you felt. It was easy for the early-stage patients to be fussy and chafe at inaction, because they didn't always feel sick. Even women who wanted to follow every rule so they could get better and get home faster had trouble staying still.

No matter whether patients were eating, reading in bed, or heading to the bathrooms, they were expected to make every movement a slow one. Lying in bed, keeping activity to a minimum, and not jostling the lungs was akin to putting a splint on a broken leg. Doctors and nurses told the women to walk with a smooth and leisurely gait when they walked at all, a movement that was universally known as "the TB glide."

Many women kept pen and paper on their bedside tables, and some expressed their feelings about chasing the cure in verse. A woman named Ruth, who was at Arequipa in the 1920s, wrote up her feelings about the rules in a poem titled "Life in a Lung Resort":

> Do not talk.
> Do not walk.
> Easy does it.
> Always sit.
> Do not stand
> Nor raise your hand
> Above your head.
> Stay on your bed.
> To cut your bill
> You must be still.[15]

Another important part of the cure was breathing the open air, because closed-in spaces like crowded homes or stuffy stores and factories were breeding grounds for TB. Arequipa was built to be a giant screened porch, so that women in their beds would feel as though they were living outside. It was not heated. This was the outdoor life in institutional form.

Living and sleeping in the fresh air might have been good for patients, but it wasn't the most comfortable way to spend days and nights. To make their beds warmer in cold weather, the women put newspapers between their mattresses and box springs. They all had hot water bottles and flannel pajamas, and for the most part they stayed cozy, at least when they were in bed. The staff, however, had to bundle up with coats and sweaters as they did their rounds.

Spending all day on the equivalent of a porch was completely counter to the way the patients normally spent their time, which was true for nearly every aspect of the TB cure. The women felt as if they were living out in the open, they ate huge meals with food they wouldn't normally have at home and had to eat it whether they were hungry or not, they had to lie down for a nap every day, and they couldn't move around the sanatorium without permission.

This sounds like a child's daily routine, and many historians have faulted sanatorium doctors for what they call the infantilization of TB patients. Susan Craddock, in *City of Plagues: Disease, Poverty, and Deviance in San Francisco*, uses Philip King Brown and Arequipa as an extreme example of this institutional control, which she calls "mapping the individual in space."[16] In her view, Dr. Brown chose Arequipa's isolated location to keep patients from wandering into nearby Fairfax and chose the architectural design of large, screened windows and open wards as a way to keep patients under constant observation.

Craddock was correct in that no one, as far as the records show, ever took an unscheduled day trip, and it was easy for nurses and doctors to see how the patients were faring from many parts of the sanatorium. But these were not Philip King Brown's original aims. Henry Bothin donated property that Brown had to alter to make building the sanatorium possible. And as we saw in chapter 5, Brown's decision to create his sanatorium as an all-in-one structure was based on cost, convenience for his staff, and the aesthetics of the land. Large windows and open wards were designed for the free flow of air, not surveillance.

Brown's paternalism did, however, show up in the "Rules and Information for Patients" that all new arrivals received. As described earlier, it was mostly a practical list of how the everyday was managed at the sanatorium. But the document also had language about attitude, which was probably the hardest part of the rest cure and one of the places where Brown exerted the most influence.

The opening paragraph of the handout introduces Arequipa's main function: curing women of TB and then teaching them how to keep from getting the disease again. Everyone was expected have the same goal, and, as Brown put it, "no patients will be kept who do not enter heartily into the spirit of the place."[17] He also made sure that patients understood that everyone from financial donors to doctors would work hard to help them and that their cooperation was expected in return.

With these ironclad rules, Dr. Brown deliberately achieved what Craddock described as disciplinary monotony: "Disciplinary monotony came in part, then, from turning the institution into the only social and experiential context of the sanatorium patient."[18] To Brown, fighting tuberculosis was a war against the disorder that created it.

The manager of any institution filled with individuals has to impose order to achieve its goals, whether it's a hospital, a school, or a business. This is why living in a sanatorium could be so hard. Women ran their children's lives by structuring their food, their sleep, and their activities. Many of them didn't like it when it was their turn.

But many women got TB in the first place because of how they lived at home or at work. To get to the medical state of "apparently cured," many had to live counter to habits they had cultivated in their home lives. This wasn't the case for everyone. But even if you lived in the cleanest, most spacious house in the world, or worked in the most modern factory, if you were exposed to someone with TB and your own health wasn't the best, you could become infected.

Most sanatoria treated both men and women, and though the sexes were kept rigidly separated, the rules were the same for both. On the surface there's something rather antifeminist about sanatorium policies; control over bodies and minds is one of the constants of women's history. But a look at the rules at Arequipa and at other tuberculosis hospitals and sanatoria demonstrates that TB did not discriminate, and neither did the treatments.

Philip King Brown felt that Arequipa was not just a place where medicine happened. It was also a place where learning happened, and where he taught the same lessons that he did in his San Francisco Polyclinic class. He had a captive audience at Arequipa, and if his rules seemed heavy-handed, it was because he knew he was in mortal combat with tuberculosis, and in his mind there was only one way to beat it back.

With dinner over, final temperatures taken, and the women reading in their beds or talking quietly with one another, the only thing left was lights out, which usually came around 9:00 P.M. After their long nap, many women found it hard to get to sleep, but as with all the other rules, bargaining and fussing were not allowed, no matter how you felt. But even if you looked forward to a long night's sleep, living in a ward with twenty or more other women did not necessarily mean that your slumber would be uninterrupted. Jackie, an Arequipa patient in the 1930s, wrote a prose poem called "Lights' Out!" about night in the sanatorium:

> Nine P.M. Lights out. The sound of snickers, a sigh and night has again descended. Here and there a faint snore ascends into the darkness, a soft whistle of gentle breathing, a heavy breathing cuts through the Ward / Sophie gasps for breath, Betty talks on and on meaningless but constant, Jo sighs loudly and startles herself, Judy snores softly. But Ella—Ella stirs the whole place with her screams. Starting softly—No—No—No— Help—Help—Help—Loudly exclaiming Get off! Get off! Get off! At last a weary—all right / We all sigh, relax and drift off again / Another day has ended at Arequipa and another Quiet? nite is well on its way.[19]

The daily routine, from waking up to meals to lights out, was the scaffolding of the TB cure. Medical treatments, which we will explore in a later chapter, were also part of this structure and served to break up the sometimes terrible monotony of sanatorium life.

Some welcome upheaval came along in May 1919. During the war, Dr. Brown put aside the upkeep of the buildings and furnishings, mostly because of cost. Everyone agreed that some renovations were needed now that the war was over, but the sanatorium's treasury was not equal to the task. Jeannette Jordan came to the rescue and paid for an astonishing array of work: new hardwood floors in the wards, dining room, and offices; new linoleum in the bathrooms and hall; fresh paint in the kitchen, bathrooms, and dressing rooms. She bought plate-glass tops for the tables in the dining room, new curtains, new light fixtures, a marble flower stand, and a floral painting by well-known local artist Alice Chittenden.[20]

There was lot going on underneath all this redecorating. Maintenance was important, of course, especially in a medical institution, and proper flooring was certainly essential. But some of the alterations the board approved and Jordan paid for went beyond necessity and into aesthetics, which has nothing to do with medicine.

Or does it? If there was anything less like a hospital, it was Arequipa, and it was already that way before the new paint, curtains, and tabletops. The attempt to make Arequipa physically pleasing had already shown results. The women who worked in the pottery, who were able to surround themselves with beauty, had measurably better outcomes. Jordan knew this and may have felt that a building full of women would appreciate the homey, pretty touches in ways that would have intangible benefits.

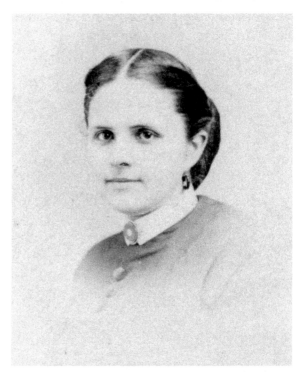

Charlotte Blake posed for this Elmira College graduation photo just before she and her
family moved to Arizona Territory in 1866. *Courtesy Elmira College Archives, Gannett-Tripp
Library, Elmira College, Elmira, N.Y.*

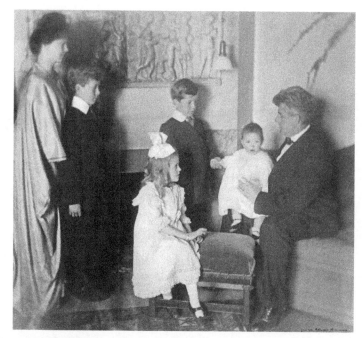

Philip and Helen Brown and their children around 1912. Hillyer stands by his mother, while Cabot, also in a dark suit, holds the hand of his little brother, Bruce. Daughter Phoebe watches her father as he holds the baby. *Courtesy Brown family.*

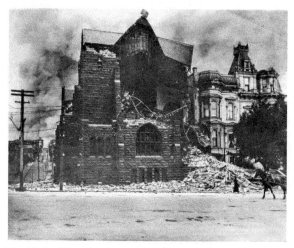

The home of Dr. Philip King Brown and his family after the earthquake of April 18, 1906, in San Francisco. The house survived the shaking, but the army dynamited it for a firebreak. *Courtesy Brown family.*

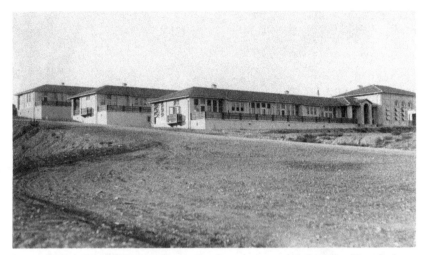

San Francisco City and County Hospital's tuberculosis ward in the 1920s. Note the large windows to allow for air circulation. *Courtesy San Francisco History Center, San Francisco Public Library.*

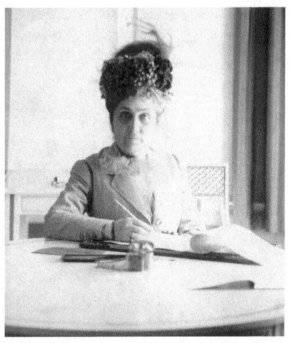

The formidable and influential Phoebe Apperson Hearst. She was a second mother to Helen Hillyer Brown and a champion of Philip King Brown's sanatorium. *Courtesy San Francisco History Center, San Francisco Public Library.*

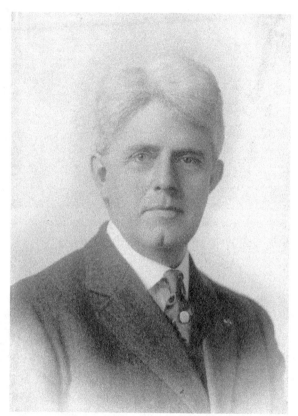

In this undated photograph, Dr. Philip King Brown echoes his mother's smile and displays the kindly demeanor that earned him the nickname "Daddy Brown" from his patients at Arequipa. *Courtesy California Historical Society.*

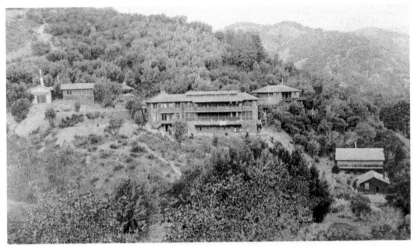

The Arequipa Sanatorium, circa 1912. The pottery shed and kiln are to the left, and out-buildings are in the right foreground. *Collection of the author.*

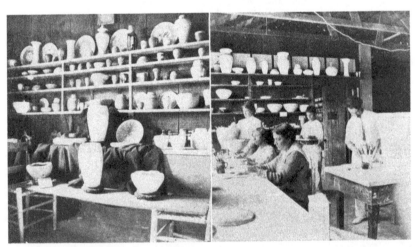

This double image appeared in annual reports beginning in 1912. On the left are pots and vases drying on shelves. On the right, pottery director Frederick Rhead supervises the patients at work. *Collection of the author.*

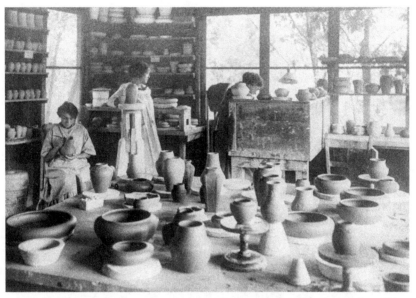

An Arequipa patient gazes out the screened window of the pottery shed as she and her fellow patients work clay, circa 1912. *Collection of the author.*

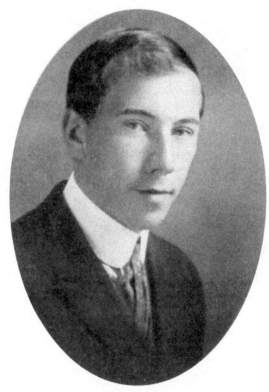

Albert Solon, Arequipa's second pottery director, in a 1918 photograph. This image appeared in *El Torre*, the yearbook of San Jose State Teacher's College, Solon's next employer after he left Arequipa. *Courtesy Tile Heritage Foundation and Jack Douglas, Librarian, Special Collections, San Jose State University.*

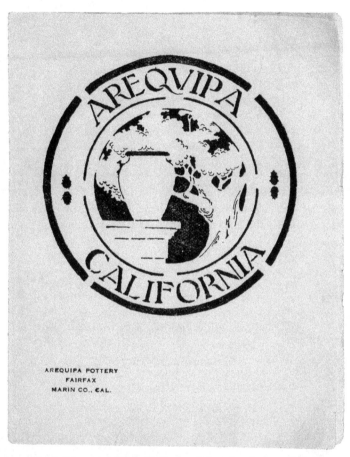

AREQUIPA POTTERY
FAIRFAX
MARIN CO., CAL.

In 1916 stores in California and beyond displayed these brochures to help boost pottery sales. Arequipa's tree-and-vase pottery mark was perfected during Fred Wilde's tenure as director and used on the newly introduced ceramic tile. *Collection of the author.*

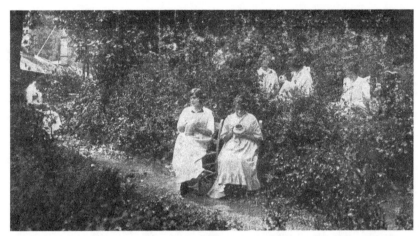

One of the chief advantages of working in the pottery was the chance to sit outdoors to carve pots and bowls. In this photo a group of patients enjoys the sun and the silence in 1912. *Collection of the author.*

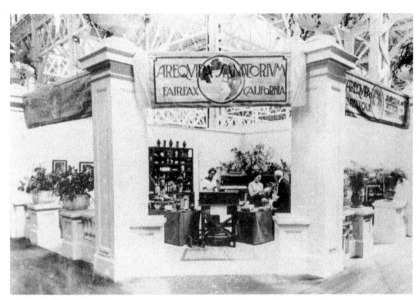

Arequipa's booth at the Panama-Pacific International Exposition in San Francisco, 1915. Visitors could watch former tuberculosis patients make pottery and could buy pieces for their own homes. Dr. Philip King Brown also used the booth to educate the public about TB prevention. *Courtesy Fairfax Historical Society Archives.*

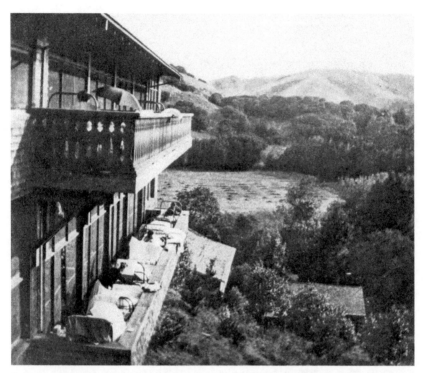

Patients who were well enough to leave their beds could sit on the outdoor balconies to take in the fresh air and the peaceful views of the Marin hills, as seen in this 1912 photo. *Collection of the author.*

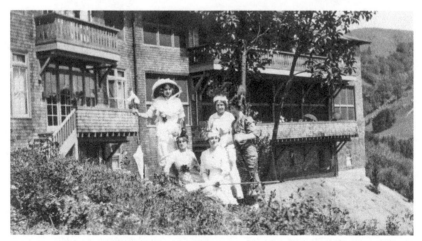

Friends and family members of Arequipa patients could drop by on specially designated visiting days. This well-dressed group posed for a commemorative photograph around 1915. *Collection of the author.*

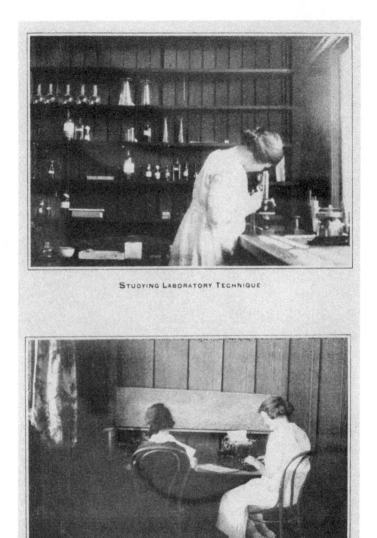

STUDYING LABORATORY TECHNIQUE

PATIENTS LEARNING TO TYPE DURING CONVALESENCE

After the pottery's demise, Dr. Philip King Brown gave his patients the opportunity to learn laboratory technology and secretarial skills, as seen in this photograph from 1924. These activities were both occupational therapy and job training to help the women navigate their post-TB lives. From the 1924 annual report. *Collection of the author.*

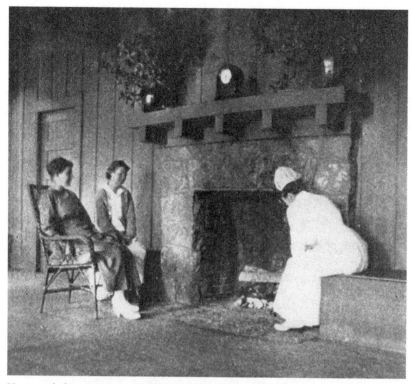

Up, or ambulatory, patients could sit by the fireplace in the living room, except at mealtimes or during the mandatory rest period. Here two patients chat with a nurse in 1912. *Collection of the author.*

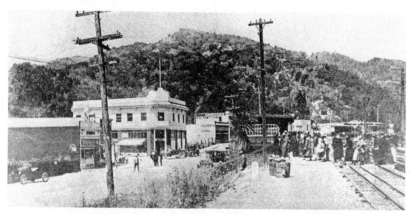

The town of Fairfax, California, circa 1925. The residents of this small West Marin city supported Arequipa by donating food and providing solace and entertainment during the sanatorium's entire lifetime. *Courtesy Anne T. Kent California Room, Marin County Free Library.*

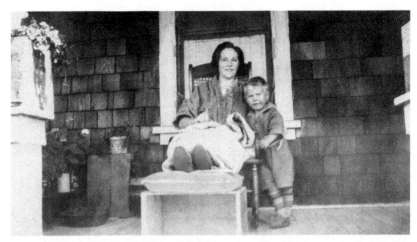

In the summer of 1927, twenty-three-year-old mother Lois Downey was diagnosed with tuberculosis. Here Lois rests on her porch with son Harvey Jr. as she tries to cure herself at home. By the fall she was worse. Her doctor would soon recommend a stay at the Arequipa Sanatorium. *Collection of the author.*

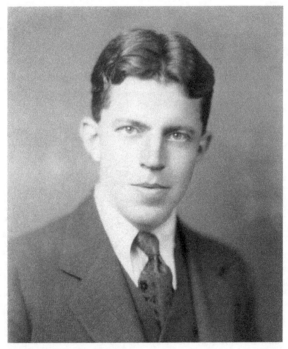

Newly minted doctor Cabot Brown, Philip King Brown's second-oldest son, joined his father's team at Arequipa and posed for this photo in 1927. He would soon be overseeing the care of a young woman from Sonoma named Lois Downey. *Courtesy Brown family.*

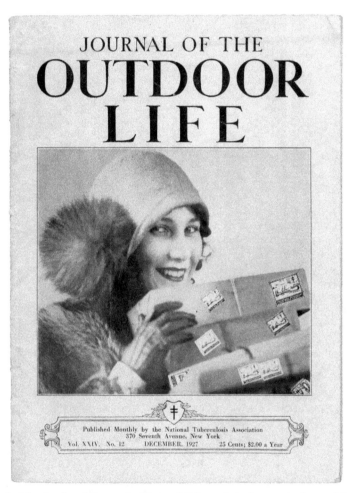

JOURNAL OF THE
OUTDOOR
LIFE

Published Monthly by the National Tuberculosis Association
370 Seventh Avenue, New York
Vol. XXIV. No. 12   DECEMBER, 1927   25 Cents; $2.00 a Year

Journal of the Outdoor Life was the National Tuberculosis Association's monthly magazine. Its articles about TB prevention were aimed at everyday Americans, not doctors. The publication also featured poetry, fiction, and advertisements for sanatoria all over the country. *Collection of the author.*

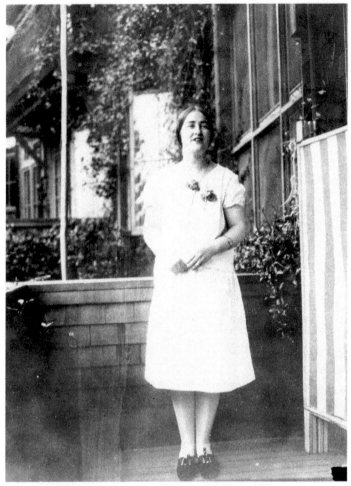

During her time at Arequipa, Lois Downey took photographs of the people who came into her orbit, and she kept them for the rest of her life. She remembered that this nurse, photographed in 1928, was a nice person but could not remember her name. *Collection of the author.*

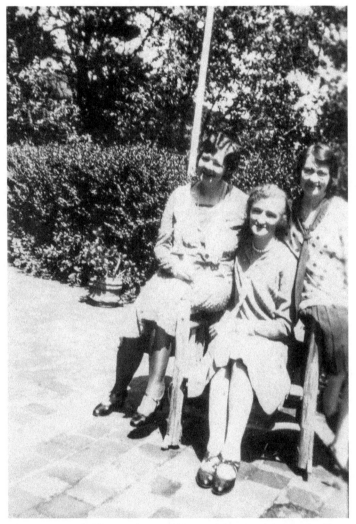

Three of Lois Downey's fellow patients—(*left to right*) Sadie, Lena, and Della—pose in their street clothes in 1929. Lena had been a nurse in nearby Santa Rosa but contracted TB and needed sanatorium treatment. *Collection of the author.*

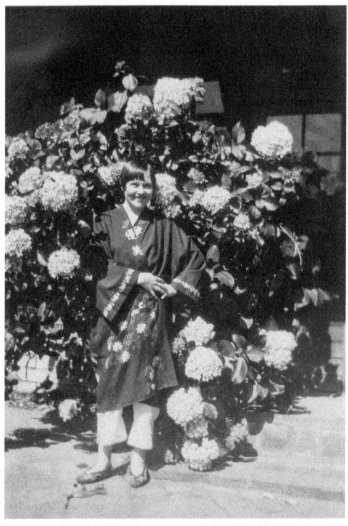

A radiant Lois Downey poses on the sanatorium's outdoor tiled patio in February 1929, after learning she would soon be discharged from Arequipa. *Collection of the author.*

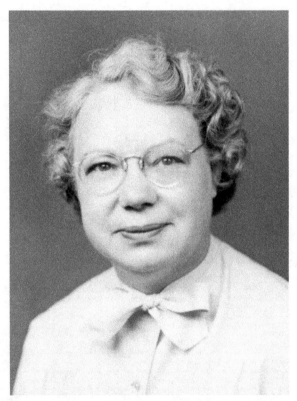

Superintendent Emma Applegren began her duties at Arequipa in 1935 and served for twenty years under the Philip King Brown and Cabot Brown administrations. She endeared herself to the patients and kept the sanatorium running during World War II, when Cabot was in the Pacific with the U.S. Naval Reserve Medical Corps. *Collection of the author.*

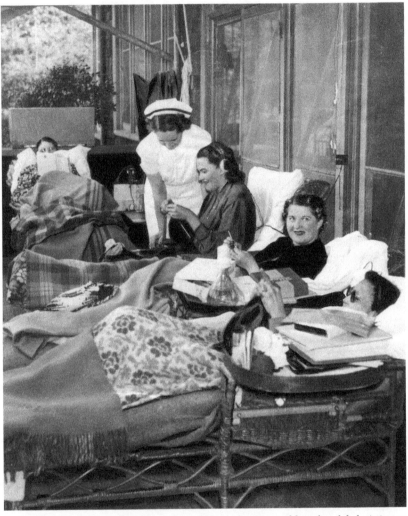

Arequipa patients spending time on the outdoor balconies could read and do knitting or other handcrafts. This photograph appeared in a *San Francisco Examiner* article, titled, "2,000 Girls Aided by Arequipa Sanatorium," on April 14, 1940. *Courtesy Anne T. Kent California Room, Marin County Free Library.*

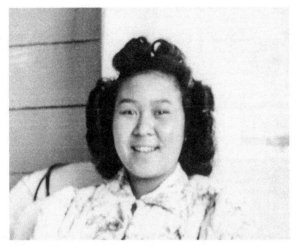

Rose entered Arequipa in June 1940 when she was just fourteen years old. Here she enjoys the sun on a patio chair while waiting to go into one of the treatment rooms. Because she was so ill, she wasn't allowed to get out of bed on her own. Two young Filipino American men carried her wherever she needed to go, a task they performed, as needed, for Arequipa's patients. *Collection of the author.*

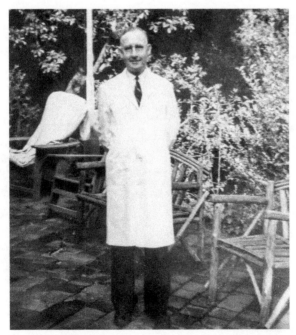

Dr. Lloyd Dickey was a pediatrician and cared for all the children taking the cure at Arequipa. He was also a visiting physician and monitored the progress of the adult patients as well. *Collection of the author.*

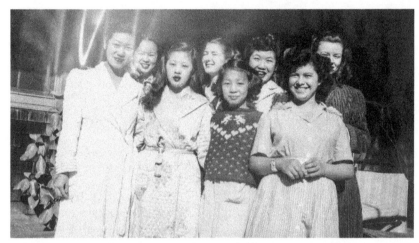

Rose stayed at Arequipa with girls and women of many races, a reflection of Philip King's and Cabot Brown's policy of nondiscrimination. In this photo from circa 1944, Rose is second from the right in the back row. *Collection of the author.*

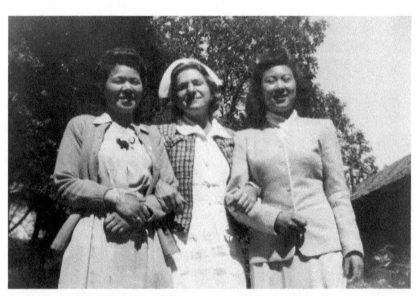

Rose made friends with both her fellow patients and the medical staff. By 1945 she was a sanatorium employee and able to get out of her robe and into fashionable clothing again. *Collection of the author.*

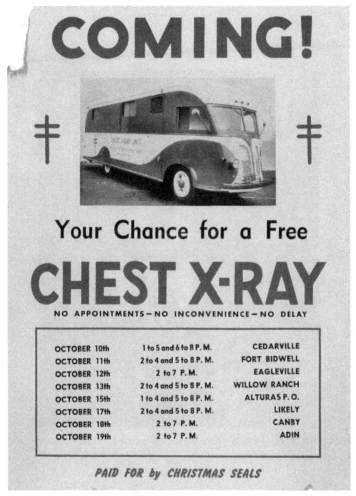

COMING!

Your Chance for a Free

CHEST X-RAY

NO APPOINTMENTS — NO INCONVENIENCE — NO DELAY

OCTOBER 10th	1 to 5 and 6 to 8 P. M.	CEDARVILLE
OCTOBER 11th	2 to 4 and 5 to 8 P. M.	FORT BIDWELL
OCTOBER 12th	2 to 7 P. M.	EAGLEVILLE
OCTOBER 13th	2 to 4 and 5 to 8 P. M.	WILLOW RANCH
OCTOBER 15th	1 to 4 and 5 to 8 P. M.	ALTURAS P. O.
OCTOBER 17th	2 to 4 and 5 to 8 P. M.	LIKELY
OCTOBER 18th	2 to 7 P. M.	CANBY
OCTOBER 19th	2 to 7 P. M.	ADIN

PAID FOR by CHRISTMAS SEALS

Mobile X-ray trucks, funded by Christmas Seals, fanned out all over California and the United States in the 1950s. This poster announced the visit of one of these units in the communities of Modoc County, in northeastern California. *Collection of the author.*

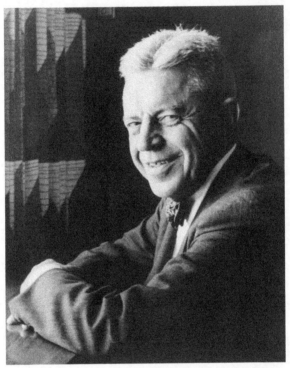

Dr. Cabot Brown in the 1950s, as he was making the painful decision to close Arequipa.
Courtesy Brown family.

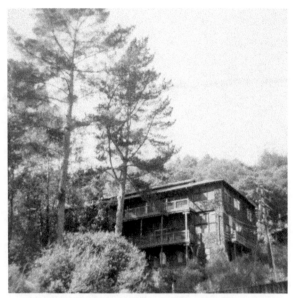

Author Lynn Downey took this photo of the empty Arequipa Sanatorium during a Girl Scout day camp outing on the property in the summer of 1965. *Collection of the author.*

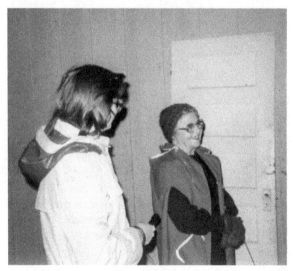

Lois Downey visits Arequipa in 1983 with granddaughter Lynn Downey. She had not been back to the sanatorium since her discharge in 1929. *Collection of the author.*

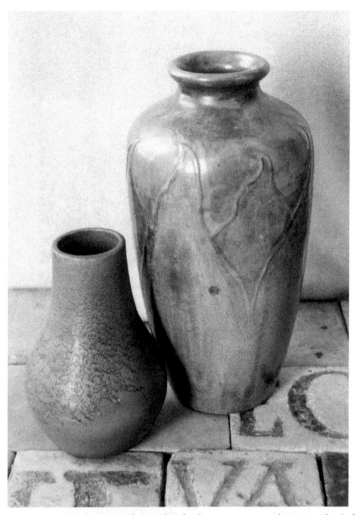

Arequipa pottery and tile are highly sought after by art pottery enthusiasts. The Oakland Museum of California and the National Museum of American History also have pieces in their collections. Individual Arequipa tiles can still be found in private collections, but installations of tiles in places such as Montecito's Casa Dorinda have generally been destroyed or paved over. *Collection of the author.*

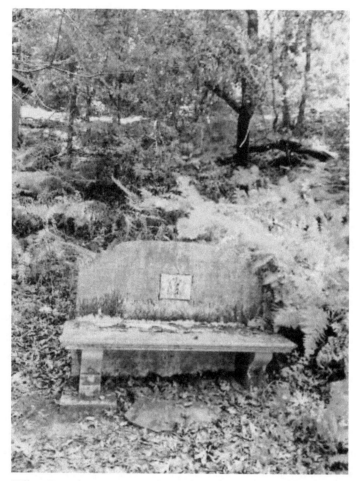

Helen Hillyer Brown's monument to her husband's work at Arequipa is this granite bench, which she installed in the early 1940s. Author Lynn Downey took this photo during her visit to Arequipa in 2015. *Collection of the author.*

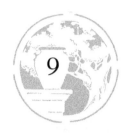

9

TO HER THE GIRLS COULD
BRING THEIR TROUBLES

SUCCESS HAD MANY FACES in the TB sanatorium world. One of them was the number of people discharged "apparently cured," but this wasn't enough for Dr. Philip King Brown. If women left Arequipa, went back to old habits, and got TB again, they were not in the ledger on the "win" side. He wanted women to go back home, or back to work, and stay healthy for the rest of their lives. To make sure this happened, he needed to follow their progress after they left Arequipa. That required social workers, and, with his usual luck, Dr. Brown found the perfect women to take on this important task.

The concept of social welfare had existed in America since before the Revolutionary War, when a combination of individual and municipal effort took care of the poor and ill. During the Civil War, the U.S. Sanitary Commission and the Red Cross emerged to add the battlefield injured to the growing list of the needy. But it was postwar industrialization—the very change that created Arequipa's working women—that saw simple caring initiatives reemerge as reform.

The settlement house was the most powerful manifestation of the new era, and from it came (mostly) women who helped create the Consumers' League, the Urban League, and the National Association for the Advancement of Colored People. Community organizing got its start in the settlement, and so did the concept of caring for individuals as "cases" and the new field of social work. The first formal social work training program was created at Columbia University in 1898, and by 1919 seventeen schools of social work dotted the country.[1]

The San Francisco Polyclinic had a Social Service Department dating back to about the time of the earthquake and fire. Since the winter of 1913, a few of its workers had been doing follow-up work with Arequipa's discharged patients, a program of special interest to Blanche Wormser, who never liked the idea of sending cured women back out into the world without checking on them afterward.

In 1915 alone the polyclinic's social service staff managed to visit between thirty and forty former Arequipa patients, and they sent out letters asking for information about the health and financial status of more than 150 others. Experienced workers were not surprised at the number of women who denied that they ever had TB, wished to forget their time at Arequipa, or resented this intrusion into their lives. Moving on was on the minds of most, and so was the desire not to be tainted with the label of former "lunger."

But there were some bright moments. Many patients returned the letters with glowing reports of improved health and employment. The polyclinic had found jobs for the husbands of a few women who were still taking it easy at home after their time at the sanatorium. Some former patients' children were now making regular trips to the polyclinic for examination and treatment too. This was good news, but sometimes the staff had to dig deeper into lives where the situation was the most desperate.

They found a pension for one widow so that she could work fewer hours per week and safeguard her health. A young woman needed treatment at Arequipa for the second time and the staff passed the hat so that she could take another cure. By the end of 1916 the polyclinic's social workers had contacted nearly all three hundred women who had taken their treatment at Arequipa since it opened and had charted their post-sanatorium progress.[2]

But having an on-site social worker was Blanche Wormser's dearest dream. She saw the need more than any of the other female benefactors, because she was the most personally involved with Arequipa. She spent a lot of time with the patients, visiting weekly and sometimes even living at the sanatorium for extended periods. Because she talked with the women, she knew what they really needed, and she gave some of the best and most prized donations of goods each year, in addition to an annual cash gift to the sanatorium's coffers.

She donated the metallic rolls for the player piano that the board of managers had given to the patients, gave each new patient a nightgown, gave each patient cash at both Thanksgiving and Christmas, and donated sewing materials, a typewriter, and prizes for the regular bridge parties. She gave auto rides to the women who were well and close to going home and donated a screen for watching movies, money for the upkeep of the X-ray equipment, and books.

Knowing the women as she did, her opinions carried weight with Dr. Philip Brown. She was very clear about how much the sanatorium needed a social worker and put her thoughts into her 1916 report to the board of managers. Arequipa needed a woman who was "inherently spiritual-minded but at the same time intelligently practical and with an abiding sense of humor," she wrote. "To her the girls could bring their troubles, individual and communal; her duties would include discovering what interests the patients have . . . that the patients may be given the opportunity of returning home better equipped for earning their livelihood or for performing their domestic duties."[3]

Her wish came true in April 1917, though she was not able to share in the good news. She had come down with an unspecified illness, and a new member of the board of managers took her place while she recuperated. This young woman would serve as secretary pro tem and then prove to be a potent force for Arequipa's social work for the next forty years. Her name was Elsie Krafft.

Like Elizabeth Ashe, Krafft was raised in comfort but took a path of service. Her father was Julius Krafft, a popular and financially successful architect. Born in Germany, Krafft arrived in Oakland in 1874 and moved to San Francisco in 1881. He opened his own architecture practice in 1888 and designed both churches and the classic Queen Anne Victorian homes that San Francisco is so famous for today.

Elsie was born in December 1875 and had one sister and two brothers. She was an intellectually precocious child. She was in the seventh grade when she was ten years old and on the honor roll of her school near the family home in the spiffy Presidio Heights district, west of downtown. After going on a tour of Europe with her father in 1894 and 1895, Elsie enrolled in the University of California in Berkeley, where she joined the Women Students' Glee Club. (She sang first alto.) She earned a degree in philosophy in 1899. In her class photo she stares straight into the camera with deep-set, dark eyes, tilting her head a bit, as if examining the photographer. Her hair is a bit messy, her dress plain, but the resolve in her face is unmistakable.

The next few years were marked by Krafft family visits to resorts all around California, even as Elsie also worked as a journalist. After women got the vote in the state in 1911, she registered as a Republican and was also involved with the Drama League of America, serving on its executive committee in 1913.

Clearly, Elsie Krafft had an affinity for the arts, but she also had a deep desire to do meaningful work. Her brothers went into the family business—Elmer was an architect; Alfred a structural engineer—but her sister, Mabel, was delicate and would later exhibit symptoms of mental illness. Elsie's character and her family's work ethic pushed her from journalism into social service, which she first undertook in 1916, the year she joined Arequipa's board of managers.

That year she was on the executive committee of the Social Workers' Alliance, which was part of the California Conference of Social Agencies. A few years earlier Krafft had joined the Social Service Department of the San Francisco Polyclinic, which is where Philip King Brown found her. He soon invited her to help undertake the formal work of tracking former patients at Arequipa. When Blanche Wormser got sick, Elsie Krafft's journalism background made her the perfect candidate to fill in as executive secretary, which she did through the end of the 1920s at least.[4] She led the follow-up work with Arequipa's patients in 1916, and in 1917 she announced in the annual report that Dr. Brown had engaged a woman named Lucy Pyle to be the resident social worker.

Lucy was born in Yreka, in the far northeastern region of California, the daughter of a shopkeeper. She formed very firm opinions early in life. In 1895, at the age of sixteen, she was among hundreds of locals who signed a petition to California state senator J. M. Gleaves, urging him to strike the word *male* from the section on voting in the California Constitution and to pass a law granting full suffrage to the women of California. The Pyle family moved to Los Angeles after the turn of the century, and Lucy's mother died in 1908. Lucy trained as a nurse in southern California and stayed there until her father's death in 1916.

She then moved up to the Bay Area and joined the polyclinic's Social Service Department, working two mornings a week in the tuberculosis clinic, screening candidates for admission to Arequipa. Though she wasn't educated as a social worker—for that matter, neither was Elsie Krafft—she got on-the-job training from the staff at the polyclinic and obviously showed an affinity for the work.[5]

Philip King Brown had a rare ability to see the potential in the people he brought into Arequipa, and didn't look at just their diplomas or their résumés. In Elsie Krafft he saw a soul devoted to service, and in Lucy Pyle a nurse whose abilities could be transferred to patient care of a different kind. Krafft and Pyle were also mature women, past their first, young learning years, and obviously had the discipline to work with TB patients of vast diversity in character and personality. Pyle was expected to help patients in all the ways that Blanche Wormser had described. The goal was to help the women live outside of their ailments and symptoms and give up behaviors that thwarted their recovery once they had finished their sanatorium treatment.

Philip Brown decided to publish more detailed information about what he and his staff had learned in their follow-up work with discharged patients, and this appeared in the 1919 annual report. In a more extensive survey, he followed 168 women from 1919 to 1922. Of these 168, 76.3 percent of the first-stage patients were healthy and working by 1922. Of the more seriously ill second and third stages, 52.6 percent were well.[6]

The report also listed what kind of jobs the women held. Stenographers and typists were the second largest group, with sixteen patients. These were followed by much smaller collections of household servants, saleswomen, clerks, trained nurses, high school teachers, factory workers, waitresses, dressmakers, children's nurses, medical missionaries, and the occasional social worker, milliner, tailor, music teacher, or dancing teacher.

The list also included a few high school and college students. But by far the women who had filled the wards in the greatest number over the previous ten years—seventy-four of them to be exact—were a surprise. They weren't sewing machine operators, clerks, or other working women who toiled in factories or stood on their feet all day in department stores.

They were housewives.

Of the twenty-seven second-stage cases on the checkup list, fourteen—just over half—were housewives. Five of these women were also the breadwinner in their family, and were described in the 1922 report: "One has supported a family of five for the past eight years and educated three children by raising chickens, rabbits and garden truck. Another takes in sewing. A third with a child and invalid mother to care for, earns their living by practical nursing. Two others divide their day between housekeeping and assisting in their husbands' business. Among the third stage cases is a star patient, the mother of nine healthy children and the head of a well-kept household."[7]

Two years later housewives were still the largest group of patients in all stages of the disease. Clearly the social workers saw wives and mothers as working women, especially the breadwinners who fell into their situation either because they were widows, had been deserted, or were married to men disabled by the conditions of their own harsh blue-collar labor.

Did Philip King Brown see them the same way? He had spent years advocating for women who went out to work, but in his early writings about the effect of TB on women's lives he frequently mentioned mothers. He obviously did not turn down any housewife who came to Arequipa for treatment, so whether or not he saw them as "workers" is irrelevant. He knew that the crowded and dark conditions of some working-class homes were as dangerous to the lungs as the dustiest textile factory.

Blanche Wormser returned to duty at Arequipa in 1919, taking on the job of treasurer instead of secretary, a less onerous task, and Elsie Krafft took up the secretary duties full-time. Blanche stayed on the scene almost to her death, which came on March 29, 1924. Philip King Brown paid her tribute in his medical director's report that year:

> Her great wish was that everything connected with Arequipa should be 100 per cent, and she spared no pains in trying to make it so. Her efforts were untiring, even during her long period of ill-health. Her loss to the Sanatorium is inestimable. Her keen interest was inspiring while she was here and will continue to be an influence during the lifetime of her fellow workers and the patients whom she befriended.[8]

After Wormser's death, her husband, Samuel, donated headphones to Arequipa so that patients could listen to radio programs without disturbing their ward mates. Wormser's life and contributions to the sanatorium stayed fresh in the minds of the doctors, nurses, and staff members, not to mention the long-term patients. They made sure the incoming women knew that an extraordinary woman had given them the radio, the movie screen, and so many other gifts. It was Blanche Wormser whose generosity helped make their treatment and their recovery a little more bearable.

After Philip King Brown got back into his postwar routine in the spring of 1919, Dr. Mary Mentzer reverted to her usual visiting physician duties. By 1921 she was teaching at Stanford, working at Arequipa, and running her own private practice. But in 1923 she realized that she needed to let something go and told Philip King Brown she had to give up her trips to Arequipa. Two other doctors were already in place in the rotation, and the loss of Dr. Mentzer caused sadness in the wards but no disruption in the sanatorium's routine.

Lucy Pyle had left Arequipa in 1920, and Elsie Krafft took over all the social service and follow-up work. And soon Dr. Ethel Owen, who had come on board as an occasional visiting doctor in 1921, took on the additional medical mantle.

Like so many of the other female physicians in Dr. Brown's sphere, she had an impressive background. She was born in Eagle Pass, Texas, in 1890, and sometime after 1900 her family moved to Los Gatos, on the peninsula south of

San Francisco. Her father died in 1909, and a few years later Ethel entered Stanford University. She got her BA in 1914 and then entered the university's medical school, one of the first female students to study medicine at Stanford. While on campus she heard Theodore Roosevelt speak about the Panama Canal. After she graduated in 1917, she began working as a medical adviser for the university's women students.

In August 1918 Dr. Owen went to France to serve as a physician with the Red Cross Children's Bureau in Paris. Organized in August 1917 under the leadership of San Francisco physician William Palmer Lucas, the bureau was dedicated to the health and rescue of the women and children of France. Lucas was a professor of children's diseases at the University of California as well and was the perfect general to manage the army of volunteer doctors and nurses, Dr. Owen among them (as well as Elizabeth Ashe, who was the bureau's chief nurse). For her service, Ethel Owen was awarded what she called a "gold medal for devotion to France"—probably the Médaille de la Reconnaissance Française. This was given exclusively to civilians who had dedicated themselves to caring for the people of France.

Dr. Owen returned to San Francisco in the spring of 1919, moving into a house with her mother and sister in Los Gatos. But she got a shock in August when her mother went into the basement and shot herself with a revolver, apparently depressed because of ill health and unspecified business troubles.

Two months later Dr. Owen was named the permanent medical adviser for women at Stanford and moved out of the family home, sharing a house with another physician in San Francisco. She worked at the state mental hospital in Napa and in May 1921 gave that up to open a private practice at 909 Hyde Street in San Francisco, which is where she met Philip King Brown, who had his office in the same building.

She began her visiting physician routine at Arequipa and balanced that with her work in the city, even after taking up Mary Mentzer's duties. But she wasn't content to rest on her medical laurels. In July 1924, at the age of thirty-four, she went to Europe to study at the University of Edinburgh and to travel around England, Switzerland, and Italy. She was gone for six months, but Arequipa's patients were well tended by a few other doctors Brown had recruited to make regular trips to the sanatorium to look after the patients, many of them men.[9]

September 1921 marked Arequipa's tenth anniversary, and Philip King Brown gave a tea at the sanatorium in celebration. Henry Bothin's wife,

Ellen, Blanche Wormser, Mary Holton, and Isabel Dibblee were in charge, and many of the founders also attended—Elizabeth Ashe, Henry Bothin, and Dr. Brown himself among them. Anyone who wanted to share in the observances could come by between two o'clock and five o'clock on Saturday, September 24.

The patients who weren't on complete bed rest helped plan the day. Holton, Wormser, and Dibblee sent flowers over on the Friday before. The ambulatory patients mixed them with some of the wildflowers growing near the building and put them in vases in the living room, dining room, and wards. The festivities started when the patients read a poem of appreciation for Philip King Brown's work and gave him a photo album of shots taken around the grounds and inside the sanatorium. Visitors enjoyed refreshments and listened to speeches, and the patients talked with returning friends who had been at Arequipa and were now enjoying good health back out in the world.[10]

Returning to Arequipa was not a threat to the revived lungs of former patients; nor was it a problem for anyone who came to the sanatorium to visit. Despite TB's easy communicability, the clean conditions in the wards and the healthful habits of the both the patients and the staff meant that anyone coming into the building was at a very low risk for picking up the bacillus. The open, screened wards took care of that too. Everyone who came to Arequipa understood this, because many of them had lived with or known TB patients themselves. Dr. Brown also made sure that patients and visitors alike knew how to conduct themselves to be safe. Arequipa schooled the healthy as well as the ill.

∾

Until the early 1920s, Arequipa's nurses were merely a white-clothed, unnamed presence in the sanatorium's board minutes and reports, revealed only occasionally as a "Mrs. Ford" or another unhelpful title. But one nurse would make herself indispensable not only to Dr. Brown but to her charges, who came to both respect and love her. She was Elizabeth Duncan MacMillan.

Born in 1874 in Dunedin, New Zealand, a southeastern coastal city full of immigrants from Scotland, she trained as a nurse in her home country and in 1913 immigrated to San Francisco, arriving in the city in August. She worked at a military academy in San Rafael and the Presbyterian Orphanage in San Anselmo (two towns just minutes from Arequipa) until about 1919, when she went back to New Zealand to visit her family.

By the spring of 1920 she was working at the Marin County Poor Farm, which was a large swath of land where the old, the ill, and the indigent were housed, fed, and given medical care. This was located in the area now called Lucas Valley, named for a nineteenth-century rancher (not filmmaker George Lucas, who built his Skywalker Ranch there). Nearby was a cemetery and a "pest house" for people with infectious diseases. Elizabeth MacMillan was listed as a servant at the farm but very likely did some nursing in addition to more mundane chores.

She was working at Arequipa by early 1922 and made quite an impression on the patients, who were soon calling her Tanta (Auntie), thanks to the sweet disposition hidden under her traditional stern nursing exterior.[11] By this time the women had a way to express how they felt about Arequipa; about having TB; about the food, the doctors, and the nursing staff. They now had their own magazine.

In 1917 Philip King Brown had asked the patients if they would like to start a sanatorium magazine, and they jumped into the project with as much vigor as they were allowed. They called it *Arequipa Gossip*, and each ward took turns editing the little paper. Writing was not only a creative activity but it was also educational and could even lead to post-sanatorium employment for women who showed aptitude with a pen or a typewriter. And under proper supervision, the work wasn't strenuous enough to interfere with lungs at rest.

Many American sanatoria had their own magazines, and their titles were either straightforward, like *Arequipa Gossip*, or were highly descriptive, such as *Grit and Grin*, published at the Firland Sanatorium in Seattle. The Peoria Municipal Tuberculosis Sanatorium had the *Peoria Fluoroscope*, the Indiana State Sanatorium's paper was the *Hoosier Res-Cuer*, the Eastern Oklahoma Tuberculosis Sanatorium published *Mountain Air*, and the J. N. Adam Memorial Hospital in New York had a different version of Firland's magazine: *Grit-Grin*.

Philip King Brown might have encouraged writing and publishing for the good it did his patients, but the women hoped it would give them a little bit of fun. Within a very short time *Arequipa Gossip* and the little magazines that followed it became vehicles for self-expression and bonding for patients.

Hi-Life succeeded *Arequipa Gossip* in September 1921. Typewritten and issued every two weeks, it dealt mostly with the health and antics of the patients in residence, news about women who had recently left, and reminders of Philip King Brown's pep talks and pet phrases. The first issue reported that many patients were learning shorthand, and the unnamed editor suggested that everyone get together at the same time to study. She ended her piece with, "As Dr. Brown says: 'Make Arequipa a school!'"

Doctors such as Philip King Brown might have hoped that in-house magazines would be uplifting, but nearly all the short items in *Hi-Life*'s columns read like the "Laughter, the Best Medicine" column of *Reader's Digest*. Many patients had nicknames, and the first issue of *Hi-Life* included a story about a Mrs. McAlpine, known as Ichabod Crane. Caught kneeling at the end of her bed and looking through the bars one night, she quipped, "Bars, and bars, but not a thing to drink." This was followed by an editorial comment: "We're sorry Ichabod, but the drinks weren't in the bargain when you came up to Arequipa."

Any progress in a patient's cure was celebrated in print, and in a way that was meaningful only to someone who understood sanatorium life. "Arequipa will soon have to ask the Board of Directors for funds to buy a special scale for the regular Friday morning weigh of Alice C.—as each time this young lady gets off the scale it has to be repaired."

Translation: Alice was getting better because she kept gaining weight.

Dr. Mary Mentzer was popular with the patients, and one women wrote up a funny exchange between the doctor and one of her charges in *Hi-Life*:

DR. MENTZER (looking at chart): "Look how fat this girl is getting."
ALICE: "Don't you think I need exercise?"
DR. MENTZER: "Yes, every Friday morning go down and get weighed."[12]

Women who were getting close to being discharged always received a few column inches. "Popular Girl Plans to Leave" and "We Hate to Lose You, Mathilda!" were typical headlines. One group of nine women went home at about the same time, and their departure was described as "leaving Arequipa Charm School."

Food was also a popular topic in *Hi-Life*. One entry read: "WANTED: By Alice A. Something to eat. Will take anything anytime. Can consume any amount, just so it is edible."[13]

Finally, there were the "Alumnae Notes," or news of former patients. "Cecelia S. has gone back to China where she is continuing to charm the natives as well as all imported humans. She's a vamp!" ran one item. "Marjorie E. has accepted a fine position in Fresno, and is now sharing the Fresno heat with the raisins," was another.[14]

Writing poetry was a popular pastime. Once the magazines came along, patients could also enjoy seeing their verse in print. As usual, the topics were about TB: getting it, getting cured of it, hoping they would get cured of it, or the sights and sounds of the sanatorium. Some poems were humorous, written either by the most optimistic patients or the ones who were about to go home.

The doctors sometimes got the poetic treatment, and in the late 1910s Philip King Brown was the subject of some humorous verse titled simply "Dr. Brown":

> When we see a piece of apple pie,
> At Arequipa San
> We know 'tis Tuesday and then we smile
> For that day a certain man
> Will come to us with his cheery way
> To encourage us all he can.
> And then at noon 'tis the apple pie
> At Arequipa San.
> To which the Doctor attention gives.
> And every Tuesday as long as he lives
> We hope he'll enjoy his pie.
> Exactly as much as you and I
> Like our splendid—
>   "Doctor Man."

The apple pie motif was repeated in 1921 in the September 25 issue of *Hi-Life*. The last two pages were filled with illustrations done by a patient named Edythe, who drew Philip King Brown in a three-piece suit, walking purposefully with a doctor's bag in his left hand and a piece of pie in his right.

But most of the poems were sad and serious, and poetry was one of the outlets for patients who tried to wear a smile but found it hard going. For some women, writing was very personal and not always meant to be shared. The contrast in purpose and topic in these verses, which many women left behind when they went home, speaks volumes about the individual path each patient was on.

A woman identified as B. C. penned a succinct piece about learning how to cure TB:

> Eat, sleep, and rest—They say is the best;
> So, if by a bug you are caught,
> This you will be taught!

And a popular patient identified as Phoebe S. wrote an eloquent poem about the place of Arequipa in her life:

> Fair Arequipa, nested in the arms
> Of ancient hills, unto whose heights I raise
> Mine eyes for help, your image, Place of Rest,
> My heart shall treasure through all coming days.

She ends the piece this way:

> Therefore I lay at your hill-encircled shrine
> My grateful heart, Oh Place of Rest, and pray
> You may endure 'til the long fight is won
> And the White Plague has lost its power to slay.[15]

MacMillan made a few appearances in *Hi-Life*, beginning in the May 12, 1922, issue:

They say experience teaches—if that is so, we're all sure Miss Macmillan can make her living from now on as a professional interior decorator! Experience? Heavens yes—three months of it, at Arequipa . . . and we must say, when a big blessing came along in the person of Miss Macmillan—then presto! The whole place nearly smiles out loud at you now! Sunshine, sunshine everywhere! What care we for cloudy days? There's sunshine on our chairs, drapes, fancy colored tins, and in our hearts! Miss Macmillan goes around, brush in hand, looking like someone who has formed a deadly habit and finds herself powerless to resist it. Clear the way! If you don't want yourself or your possessions painted, put them under lock and key. As for the best nurse that ever was—we're thinking of tying a ball and chain to her, so as not to run the risk of ever having her escape.

This issue also had a drawing of a patient with a bandage on her finger standing next to a woman in a nurse's uniform and cap, paintbrush in hand, with the caption "*Mildred:* Hey! Miss MacMillan. I wish you would fix my finger. *Miss McMillan:* I wish you wouldn't bother me. This is more important than your finger."[16]

Ethel Steeves was a stern superintendent, but she wasn't so strict that she created a barrier between herself and the patients, and this comes out in their writing. In the September 25, 1921, issue of *Hi-Life*, a column titled "Captain

Back! Ship Ahoy!" reported on Steeves's return to Arequipa after taking a holiday: "There was probably nothing that added more to the joy of Arequipa's girls than to have Miss Steeves back again after her vacation in Honolulu. Miss Baker filled in her absence to a great extent. She's such a good old sport, that no one can help loving her,—but of course there's only ONE Miss Steeves. We're mighty glad to have her with us again."

This issue included drawings by the artistic patient Edythe, and Ethel Steeves was also one of her subjects. The top of the page featured a bathing-suit-clad woman sitting on a beach next to a palm tree with the words "Miss Steeves" underneath and "On the beach at Wai-ki-ki" as the drawing's title. Above her head was a cartoon thought bubble and inside it a drawing of a building surrounded by trees and captioned "Arequipa."[17]

On April 21, 1922, the patients threw Ethel Steeves a surprise birthday party. After morning weigh-ins and temperature taking, she tactfully drove away to do some errands so that the patients could ready the sanatorium for the event. (They could not possibly manage a surprise party without her cooperation and approval, and the patients had already given her full details about their plans.) When she came back, all the patients—even the bed-bound ones—were dressed as characters from *Alice in Wonderland*, who formally introduced themselves one by one as Steeves sat in the dining room to receive them. There followed a lovely dinner, which Ethel Steeves had personally selected: asparagus salad, broiled chicken, and ice cream. Between courses the healthiest patients acted out scenes from the book, and the White Rabbit, after hunting all over the dining room for her white gloves, handed them to Steeves as a birthday present. A cake with twenty-one candles (for the day of the month, not her age) was then wheeled in and everyone got a piece.[18]

What does this tell us? That MacMillan was loved and respected enough that patients could make fun of her without risk. The same goes for Steeves, who shared the details of her personal life with her charges. This is something rare. Nurses were trained to be dispassionate about their patients and not allow their feelings to interfere with the job. They could not have any "dreaming time," as one nurse put it in an 1890 newspaper interview. If they took on the troubles that confronted them every day, they would crumble.[19] But this does make sense. Unlike a hospital, where a nurse would have charge of patients for just a few days or perhaps weeks, the women of Arequipa saw MacMillan every day for months or years. One would have to be the most hardened nurse ever trained to not find herself moved by the plight and the playfulness of her charges.

Philip King Brown was lucky in his medical staff. They shared many attributes in common, not the least of which was a dedication to their profession that overrode its many hardships. They also had inexhaustible energy. Despite holding multiple positions in universities and hospitals on top of their work at Arequipa, doctors found time to make the long trip to western Marin County and back to their domestic and professional bases in San Francisco. The nurses lived together in a small cottage on the grounds, apparently forgoing much of a social life except on their days off. These were commitments of incredible depth.

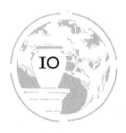

IO

PLEASANT DIVERSIONS,
UNPLEASANT TREATMENTS

HAVING THE PROPER FRAME OF MIND was near the top of Philip King Brown's list of how to get cured of TB, right after the mandate to live the outdoor life. This meant that the women at Arequipa were expected to get along with each other, but he didn't tell them how that was supposed to happen.

He read many articles about sanatorium life in medical literature and popular magazines, and most doctors shared Brown's attitude. Taken together, these articles make it clear that the women, despite their dependent state, were pretty much responsible for their own cure. They had to follow the rules, endure the medical treatments without complaint, and make sure to live appropriately when they went home (also, no spitting). Hardly anyone wrote about the emotional cost of TB treatment, except to say that patients should not dwell on negative thoughts. Social workers took a different approach though. They studied the mental attitudes of people in sanatoria and classified them by attitude: hopeless, rebellious, worried, reasonable, and so on.

The patients directed these attitudes at their medical treatments, the doctors and nurses, or the routine in general; that is, at the individual experience of sanatorium life in a communal setting. Many women had been in a hospital on occasion, but time there was usually limited to a few days or a week. A sanatorium stay had no expiration date, and in Arequipa's first decades, all patients were lumped together in the wards no matter what level of disease they had. A patient who still coughed up blood might be in a bed next to one who was just days from going home and was no longer contagious.

This was probably a function of how small Arequipa was. Municipal sanatoria could be the size of a major city hospital, making it easier to separate patients according to illness. But Dr. Brown didn't have that luxury, even with a new wing. So patients were essentially in the same boat and expected to react to their cure the same way, no matter how different their physical or mental condition was. Some doctors, however, did not think that people of different disease stages and social classes should be grouped together.

Dr. Charles L. Minor of Asheville, North Carolina, was a TB specialist and former president of the National Association for the Study and Prevention of Tuberculosis. In 1918 he wrote an article titled "The Psychological Handling of the Tuberculous Patient." Among the many pages of advice for dealing with patients who were nearly always gloomy and unwilling to follow rules was his firm belief that patients of different social classes should not be in wards together. Especially female ones. "While social selection of patients is most difficult and can only be carried out to a limited degree, it is very important," he wrote. "Mrs. Social Leader will not mix with Mrs. Ordinaire easily or naturally, though men are better about this, and where mutual scorn or resentment exists the creation of a proper atmosphere is impossible."[1]

Despite his own lofty social class, Philip King Brown did not look at his sanatorium this way. When a woman was admitted to Arequipa, she was put in the first available bed, no matter who was in the one next to her. This could have been because Arequipa's early patients were all working-class women, but there were hierarchies within even this category. The secretary to a captain of industry was a wage-earning woman, but so was the woman who sewed the clothes the secretary wore, and they could easily be ward mates. Brown never considered separating the poor from the economically comfortable.

This brings us again to the topic of race.

When a sanatorium advertised for patients but did not want people of color, the director did not hesitate to say that the beds were for whites only. Cities and individual doctors opened some sanatoria specifically for African American and Native American tuberculars, since they weren't welcomed elsewhere. This is not a surprise, but Arequipa was one of the exceptions.

Among the many examples Dr. Charlotte Brown set for her children was an unwillingness to succumb to the race prejudice of her day. In San Francisco that meant that she treated Chinese women. She also operated a dispensary in conjunction with the Methodist Episcopal Church's Chinese Domestic Mission in Chinatown, an organization that helped women find their way out of prostitution, one of many similar groups that operated in late nineteenth-century San Francisco.

In 1883 Charlotte published a paper about her work, titled "Obstetric Practice among the Chinese in San Francisco," in the *Pacific Medical and Surgical Journal*. She noticed that when a woman was having a difficult labor and wanted the help of a doctor, she (and her husband) would allow only a female physician to come to the bedside, and this usually meant a white one. And though Charlotte made some fairly typical comments about "the Chinese" as a culture apart from her own, she did not think these patients deserved anything less from her or any other doctor.

Though Philip King Brown kept the administrative side of Arequipa white, many of the patients were women of color, and this was true for the sanatorium's entire forty-six-year lifetime.

Nothing in the annual reports, advertising, newspaper articles, or Philip King Brown's own writings says anything about Arequipa being restricted. Historical records and photographs (as well as my interviews with former patients) demonstrate that Asian American and African American women were welcomed, though there are no records to indicate if indigenous women ever applied to enter Arequipa. And just like women of varying social classes, the women of color were not segregated from the white patients.

The annual reports, which are very detailed about the number of women treated and which occasionally list patients' occupations, never used racial descriptions. The few surviving medical records do list the races of the women who were admitted, but that indicates thoroughness not racism. (Think of the forms we fill out today that ask for the same information.)

Dr. Brown's policy went against convention for pre–World War I San Francisco. The D. W. Griffith film *The Birth of a Nation* debuted in the city in 1915, outraging black citizens and those opposed to racial oppression. Local political and reform leaders organized protests against the movie even as the Ku Klux Klan applied for a charter in California.[2] Chinese emigration was stymied or at least reduced to a trickle after the passage of the 1882 Chinese Exclusion Act, which was supported by the majority of Californians.

The medical director of any sanatorium could have easily kept nonwhites out of the institution. As it happens, no other California sanatorium had stated discriminatory policies in 1911, at least those that advertised in the National Tuberculosis Association's directory of that year. Dr. Brown could have set racial limits if he'd wanted to and no one would have called him names, but there is no evidence that he did.

~

Philip King Brown believed in right thinking; perhaps this was the source of his policy not to discriminate when it came to medical care. His emphasis on always staying positive, on having right thinking as an integral part of the TB cure, could be exhausting for his patients, however. Brown knew this, so he and his staff worked hard to fill the women's hours with entertainment as well as the useful occupations of pottery or magazine publishing. They could keep themselves busy with approved activities such as reading or light sewing, but bringing in a variety of outside entertainers went a long way toward getting women to that important positive state of mind.

Pleasant distraction was already a sanatorium staple. Dr. Edward Trudeau had brought in outsiders to his Adirondack Cottage Sanitarium for years. Medical journals frequently featured articles about the value of amusements in helping patients forget themselves. To make this happen at Arequipa, Philip King Brown talked to his friends and donors once again.

In 1912 someone donated a Victrola to the sanatorium, and a collection of phonograph records came in soon after. Books and magazines arrived by the dozens, not only from individuals but also from local libraries. For Christmas of 1912, the musical instrument company Sherman & Clay of San Francisco loaned Arequipa a portable organ so the women could sing carols. Another donor arranged for the occasional loan of a movie projector. These kindnesses were repeated year after year, and Philip King Brown also tapped into the talents of his friends to provide live entertainment. The sanatorium had a piano in the dining room, and either a visitor, nurse, or ambulant patient played sprightly tunes as young women from local towns came by to demonstrate the latest dance steps.

By 1919 these varied activities were gathered together under an umbrella called the Amusement Bureau, managed by Charles W. Carruth. He was a printer, publisher, and poet from Oakland and took on the bureau as his personal contribution to the cause. An article in the *Oakland Tribune* said that Carruth " has booked many high-class attractions" for the sanatorium.[3] It's not surprising Philip King Brown knew someone with the creative reach to pull together an interesting mix of talented people willing to go out to Arequipa.

Dr. Brown was very grateful to Carruth and to the people who made such an effort.

"Into the narrow life of the wards, these generous artists bring a freshening breeze from the world of music, literature and science," he wrote in 1922.[4] During 1920 and 1921 alone the patients were entertained by people renowned all over California, as well as those well-known only to the local community, but all of them were welcomed. Singers were always on the list, either singly or in groups, but Carruth looked beyond the conventional for the Amusement Bureau.

Professor E. O. James, from the women-only Mills College in Oakland, read O. Henry stories to the patients. Charles Keeler was an author, ornithologist, and naturalist who was also deeply committed to the ideals of the Arts and Crafts movement. He gave a lecture on birds and also read some of his poems. In fact, birds and nature in general seem to have been very popular topics.

Mrs. D. W. De Veer, a curator at the Oakland Public Museum, gave an illustrated talk on birds. Lillian Lamoureux, who called herself Loriol M. Vernet Lamoureux, was nationally known as "the bird philosopher" and had an enormous avian menagerie at her home. Her early life is murky, but by around 1920 she was living in Berkeley and going into hospitals and TB sanatoria telling bird stories. She always brought along her favorite robin, named Cheer. In 1920 or 1921 she visited Arequipa to give a lecture on birds, but whether Cheer came with her was not mentioned in the Amusement Bureau section of the annual reports.

Gertrude Williamson spent a month at Arequipa during the summer of 1921, staying in one of the cottages on the property reserved for the occasional overnight guest. She was a teacher at the Santa Barbara State Teachers College, which later became a campus of the University of California. Philip King Brown's connections in Santa Barbara helped him find Williamson, whose talks on nature lore and gentle nature walks (for the women allowed to do more than glide) were very popular. She even held a contest and awarded a colorful calendar as a prize to the patient who could name the most local trees.

But the most unusual entertainer was Esther Birdsall Darling. Born into wealth in Sacramento, she was raised in the family mansion there and on the Birdsall ranch in the Sierra Nevada town of Auburn, along with a vast menagerie of lost or injured animals that her kind-hearted mother gathered up and cared for. These included not only cats and dogs but also a lamb, a turtle, a blue jay, and, strangely, a monkey. Esther grew up loving both animals and reading, as her family kept quantities of books on hand in both of their homes.

She went to Mills College and in 1907 married Charles Edward Darling, who ran an expedition outfitting company in Nome, Alaska. The couple moved to

Alaska, and there Esther Darling became fascinated with the sled dogs used to haul commercial goods. In 1908 she and her husband's partner, Scotty Allen, founded the Nome Kennel Club and established Alaska's first long-distance sled dog races. They also had their own kennel, and the Darlings and Allen had a team led by a dog named Baldy.

In 1913 Esther Darling began to write a series of dog novels, beginning with *Baldy of Nome*. When the United States entered World War I, the government commissioned the Darling and Allen kennel to provide dogs for war service: carrying supplies over mountain terrain between France and Germany. Some of them were the descendants of Baldy himself. And in June 1917 France awarded Esther Darling the Croix de Guerre for the services her dogs provided to the nation.

By 1920 Darling was living in Berkeley and spoke around the Bay Area about her novels and about Alaskan sled dogs. In November 1920 she appeared at Paul Elder's bookstore in San Francisco to tell stories of the Far North and about dogs in literature. Not only that, the advertisement for her lecture included an additional enticement: "Baldy will be present."

Birdsall was a local celebrity, so Dr. Brown asked her to come to Arequipa to entertain the patients in late 1920. She gave a lecture titled "Talks on Alaskan War Dogs," though Baldy, unfortunately, was not invited. As with Cheer, animals were not especially welcome at Arequipa, though the staff tolerated the occasional cat because they kept the mouse population down.

Philip King Brown thought the radio was a good form of distraction and relaxation for his patients, but some of his fellow physicians did not agree. Dr. William H. Rosenau, a Johns Hopkins–trained doctor who practiced in the southern California town of Banning in the early 1920s, thought the radio did have its place, but it wasn't for everyone. Straining their ears to find a station or listening to melodramatic radio plays sometimes left patients "nervously overwrought, unable to sleep, and greatly excited," he wrote in a 1926 article. This led to a rise in temperature or pulse, which were indications of TB activity in the body.

To prove his point, he cited a study undertaken at the Cragmor Sanatorium in Colorado Springs during the 1925 World Series, when the Pittsburg Pirates defeated the reigning champion Washington Senators in seven games. Patients who were interested in the outcome of the game but did not listen to the radio had no untoward symptoms. Twenty-five percent of the patients who did listen to the games on the radio were examined and had no adverse reaction, but they tended to be those whose TB was already under control and who were close to being discharged from Cragmor. However, 75 percent of those who followed the games had "unfavorable" reactions, which the sanatorium's staff traced directly to the excitement of the competition. Rosenau's conclusion: each patient should be evaluated about the tendency to get overexcited before being allowed to use a radio.[5]

Not all activity was intended to be amusing. Most sanatoria, Arequipa included, brought in clergymen on Sundays to give spiritual comfort to the patients. Different denominations came at varying times, but a preacher came by each week to give short sermons in Arequipa's living room for the women who were allowed to get out of bed.

Then there were the lectures. Philip King Brown's revolving staff of visiting physicians gave the occasional educational talk in the living room, and anyone who wasn't completely bed-bound and running a high temperature could attend. The topics were always about tuberculosis: how to maintain the sanatorium's sanitary conditions when patients went home, how to continue living the outdoor life, and the importance of the proper attitude in preventing a relapse.

Doctors expected patients to change the way they lived, which sometimes included how they dressed. Anything that restricted breathing was not healthy, no matter how socially acceptable it was. When Arequipa opened in 1911, some women were still wearing corsets. Physicians had long tried to get older women to give up their corsets, both the old-fashioned lace-up kind and the newer elastic versions. This was generally a losing battle, and doctors sometimes just had to wait until the corset went out of fashion.

The 1920s saw the emergence of a new enemy. The cultural rifts of World War I created an opening for women to increase their demands for the vote, to reach for new freedoms, and to aspire to work not just for a wage but to fulfill personal ambitions. At the same time, another "new woman" was emerging: the flapper. She usually didn't have to work, as many of the women who could afford this lifestyle had money of their own. They were sexually independent and very single. Working women aspired to their glamorous nightlife, but often the only thing they could do was emulate some of their less healthy habits.

During the Gatsby era, sanatorium lecture topics often included finger-wagging about the flapper. Women smoked and dieted to achieve the thin, flat-fronted form that was now showing up in magazines and films, which was exactly how they should *not* live if they wanted to prevent TB. And while some conservatives railed against the decade's rising hemlines, Philip King Brown was not one of them. In 1922 he gave a very succinct quote on the subject to the *San Francisco Chronicle:* "Short skirts do not sweep up germ-laden dirt from the streets. In that way they are an aid in the prevention of disease."[6]

Whether listening to lectures, singers, or the radio or simply reading in bed, Arequipa's patients were expected to keep a grip on their emotions, obey all the rules of the cure, and make at least a pretense of getting along with the other women. Emotions aside, Arequipa was a pleasant place to spend your time. It was physically beautiful and sat in a wooded and quiet little valley, and even though daily life was regimented and monitored, spending a few months there wasn't so bad. Many other sanatoria were more hospital-like, with bilious paint on the walls, few windows, and fewer views. So, from a visitor's perspective, a sanatorium stint could be a lot worse.

But these people were forgetting something. Everyone they came to see, and all the women in the beds next to their wives, sisters, and friends had a lurking fear behind every smile.

Death.

～

The whole purpose of spending time at Arequipa was to fight off death. A woman might have an early-stage case of tuberculosis, but that didn't mean it was a "slight" case of TB, like a slight cold. Left untreated, small tubercles became big ones, and a sanatorium stay became less effective. But even the rest cure wasn't really a cure. Every day in your bed was a struggle, and if death came for one of your friends down the ward, you could grieve, but you couldn't forget how easily TB could take you too.

The occasional passing demoralized the patients, and this is why doctors like Philip King Brown usually didn't take more seriously infected women into their sanatoria. The rest cure was rarely effective for them, and if they died, the effect on the other patients was devastating and was a barrier to the positive outlook they were supposed to keep each day.

The daily routine, the food, and the TB glide were the main barriers against death, and the medical staff were the gatekeepers. The patients knew this and were grateful for it, caring deeply for particular physicians or nurses whose attentions seemed to make the most difference in their own lives. A smile, a conversation, and a good bedside manner were not all the doctors brought to Arequipa. Some women needed additional treatments to push their cure forward, and it is remarkable to realize that their warmth and gratitude were still intact even after enduring medical interventions that ran the gamut from the uncomfortable to the truly horrifying.

Philip King Brown kept up to date on all the new treatments being used in other sanatoria and tried a few of the more experimental ones at Arequipa. But he was also a traditionalist, and when it came to lungs, he started with X-rays.

In 1895 German mechanical engineer Wilhelm Roentgen discovered the X-ray, so-called because in mathematics X indicates something unknown, and Roentgen at first didn't know where the radiation came from. Doctors quickly realized that an X-ray was the perfect diagnostic tool for tuberculosis work. Properly done, the X-ray picture showed tuberculous lesions in the lungs even before a patient showed symptoms, though the machines could not easily distinguish between healed and unhealed lesions or detect the disease's very early stages. But it was still one of the best ways to get a jump on treating the individual sufferer, and Philip King Brown insisted on seeing an X-ray plate before admitting any woman to Arequipa.

Potential patients could get their test from any physician, but Philip King Brown had contracted with Dr. Anna Davenport to do the work specifically for Arequipa. Born in Michigan around 1871, she earned her medical degree from the Medical College of South Carolina State University. She spent some time in Hartford, Connecticut, and interned at the New England Hospital for Women and Children in Boston. By 1910 Charlotte Brown's hospital for women and children had caught her eye and she moved to San Francisco to intern there. Two years later she was a teaching assistant in surgery at the University of California Medical School.

Dr. Davenport had an office a few blocks from the one where Philip King Brown worked, and she donated her time and the cost of the plates to Brown's work. Even if a woman had an X-ray from her own physician, Dr. Davenport also took some pictures, so that Brown could verify what other doctors had diagnosed. He then also had a baseline for every patient.

Dr. Davenport began to work with Arequipa's patients in 1912 and continued to provide X-ray services through 1914, when she resigned her teaching position at the University of California. She was also working in the dispensary at Mount Zion Hospital in San Francisco, but in 1917 she moved to New York to further her career there. Dr. Brown said her great skill was essential to getting the early cases into Arequipa, where they had the best chance of recovery.

Seeing how important the machinery was to the TB cure, Mary Raymond donated X-ray equipment to Arequipa in 1915. Philip King Brown still used Dr. Davenport's services in San Francisco for women who needed treatment at Arequipa, but he also hired women to work the machines at the sanatorium itself so that patients could get regular chest X-rays.

He brought in women who were not doctors and who had no previous training in the field. This was not unusual. When doctors started buying X-ray equipment for their offices, they soon realized that the process of taking and developing the images and maintaining the machines was tedious and time-consuming. They had to turn these tasks over to someone else, and those someones were usually their office assistants, even the receptionists, meaning that some of the earliest radiology technicians were women. This was especially true after 1916 when many men were in Europe fighting in the Great War. This hole in the practice of medicine gave some women an unexpected new career.

To keep up with his X-ray program, Philip King Brown hired a young college graduate named Hazel White to run the machines. Born in San Francisco in 1892, she had demonstrated a facility for solving puzzles when she was a child and had graduated from high school in San Mateo, south of the city, in 1911. She then studied chemistry at Stanford University and was a founder of the Alchemia sorority there in 1913. She looked younger than her years in yearbook photos, with a round face, full cheeks, and a slight, serious smile.

White graduated with a BA in chemistry in 1915 and by 1916 was doing radiology work at Arequipa. How she got her training is a mystery, though Brown may have sent White to Dr. Anna Davenport's office. Recognizing her chemistry skills, Dr. Brown also hired her to assist the nurses on microscopic studies of the patients' sputum to evaluate the differences between early- and later-stage infections.

Hazel White continued her work at Arequipa into 1917. She then got engaged. While planning her wedding, she contracted influenza during the great postwar flu epidemic and died on January 1, 1919. She was just twenty-six years old.

The other "radiologist" Philip King Brown asked to work at Arequipa was Louisiana Scott Foster, a Marin County native and related by marriage to the Kittles, Isabel Dibblee's family. She was a debutante who, with no nursing training, volunteered to take care of local soldiers felled by the 1918 flu, roared around Marin in her own car, survived a deadly local train crash, and scorned marriage for work and travel.

Louisiana joined the staff at Arequipa in 1921 as a volunteer radiographer, and Philip King Brown praised both her and her work ethic. He knew he couldn't keep her forever, but he was grateful that she donated her time "to the cause," his favorite phrase.

Brown was always looking for the best interventions for TB care, and in 1916 he started using another common treatment: pneumothorax (collapse of the lung), whose name combines the Greek *pneumo*, meaning "lung" or "air," and the Greek *thorax*, meaning "chest."

In the eighteenth-century, physicians in France noticed that when some patients suffered a spontaneous collapse of a tubercular lung, they started to improve. No one understood why, but by around 1888, Italian physician Carlo Forlanini had developed a way to induce artificial pneumothorax by injecting nitrogen into the pleural cavity around the lung, causing it to collapse. The procedure made its way to America before the turn of the century.

Dr. Edmond R. Long, who worked at Dr. Edward Trudeau's Saranac Laboratory in 1919, described its usefulness in TB treatment in medical journals. "The idea back of the procedure is the same as that back of bed rest or of lying, day in, and day out, in a reclining 'cure chair,'—functional rest, enforced rest of the affected part," he wrote. In other words, it was like putting a splint on the lung, forcing it to stop moving. Dr. Long also compared a tubercular lung to an infected cut on the palm of the hand. "What are the chances of first-intention healing if that hand is opened and shut twenty thousand times a day?"

He also illustrated how the infected lung could spread "scattered groups of soft cheesy tubercles" throughout the body when the lung is not resting. "Let us remember the countless minute drainways, the lymph channels, leading away from the neighborhood of these tubercles and all other parts of the lung, forming a vast interlacing system, with the contained lymph ebbing and flowing, forward and backward, more or less in response to the lung's expansion and retraction."[7]

Philip King Brown used pneumothorax on patients who weren't improving: the ones who didn't gain weight, whose temperature stayed high, or whose X-rays showed that the lesions in their lungs were still large and not healing over. This treatment was not something the women looked forward to, and though doctors called it artificial pneumothorax or collapse therapy, patients called it "getting gas."

The pneumo apparatus itself was small: a foot-tall cylinder inside a box was connected to a hose with a large needle at the end. The cylinder was full of sterile nitrogen gas, and a nurse (or sometimes a doctor) would insert the needle into a patient's back, going through the ribs and into the pleural cavity of the diseased lung. The nitrogen would then get pumped into the pleura, causing the lung to collapse like a popped balloon. The needle was removed and the patient was taken gently back to her bed.

After this treatment, patients generally felt short of breath, as if they had a weight on their chest. They also had pain for a while, but as the gas gradually left the body, these symptoms diminished. They were instructed how to move—or rather how not to move—to make sure the collapse was doing its job.

Just one pneumo might give a patient the push she needed to move toward improvement. But most women got regular gas injections, and this could lead to complications, such as pleural embolism, shock, or sepsis. But these were rare.

In the early 1920s, new surgeries were also making the rounds at sanatoria, and many were used on Arequipa patients, but not at the sanatorium itself. Sometimes adhesions or scars formed between the pleural cavity and the lung, preventing the gas from doing its work. When this happened, doctors had to remove the adhesions in a procedure called a pneumolysis.

Advanced cases called for more drastic measures, such as collapsing the lung permanently. This meant a thoracoplasty: removing some ribs on one side of the chest, a procedure that induced more dread than any other.

These were serious surgeries, so when Philip King Brown's patients needed them, his colleagues at the Cottage Hospital in San Rafael or at San Francisco General took on the task. After a short recuperation, the women went back to Arequipa and their treatment continued. If the adhesions were gone, they could get gas. After thoracoplasty, the women simply had to make sure they stayed quiet. They then learned to live with a lung that would never be whole, a life of half breath.

Everyone knew when a woman had to leave the sanatorium for surgery, and most departures were covered in the sanatorium magazine. In September 1921, an article in *Hi-Life* titled "Popular Young Lady Undergoes Successful Operation" reported on Frances C., "better known as Buck," who returned to Arequipa from San Francisco. "She looks 'Pale Budweiser' and here's hoping that she will get back all the lost pounds soon."[8]

By the mid-1920s, Arequipa also had a fluoroscope machine, thanks to a generous and anonymous donor. The fluoroscope took the same kind of image as an X-ray but in real time; that is, the patient stood behind an illuminated screen that revealed the body's inner workings as she breathed. (The technology was shown in old-time cartoons as animated human and animal characters watching their bouncing skeletons exposed on a screen.)

The two systems worked best in tandem. While the X-ray was better at detecting tubercular lesions early on, the fluoroscope was best for routine examination of lung tissue. By the mid-1920s the fluoroscope ruled at Arequipa.

Dr. Brown looked beyond the conventional, whether in people or TB treatments. In March 1921 the National Tuberculosis Association gave $4,000 to the Hooper Foundation for Medical Research in San Francisco to investigate the potential healing properties of something called chaulmoogra oil.

The Hooper Foundation was chartered in 1913 with an endowment from the widow of George Williams Hooper, a San Francisco lumber merchant and philanthropist. It was the first medical research foundation in the United States affiliated with a university—in this case, the University of California. Dr. Ernest L. Walker, a specialist in tropical diseases, was hired to conduct studies to see if oil from the chaulmoogra tree might kill the TB bacillus.

His experience in tropical medicine was important. The oil, from a tree native to East India, had been used for centuries as a treatment for leprosy, and modern doctors found that it actually worked with many of their leprosy patients. The TB bacillus had a similar structure to the one that caused leprosy, and this was intriguing to doctors. They thought chaulmoogra oil's antibacterial and antiseptic qualities might give them a weapon against TB. The oil was also known in popular culture. It was featured in the 1924 Agatha Christie novel *The Adventure of the Egyptian Tomb* and was an important plot point that helped detective Hercule Poirot solve an archaeologist's murder.

In the spring of 1921, Philip King Brown got in touch with the Hooper Foundation and offered up Arequipa patients as test subjects for Dr. Walker's investigation into chaulmoogra oil. Between June and December, Walker came by regularly and injected a solution of the oil into the muscles of seventeen patients, but they didn't show any improvement, no matter how long Walker waited for results. Philip Brown later wrote that there seemed to be some improvement in the women who had tubercular laryngitis, enteritis (intestinal inflammation), and empyema (a bacterial infection in the pleural cavity around the lung), but the experiment didn't last long enough or undergo enough follow-up to be considered a success. Tuberculosis doctors eventually decided that chaulmoogra oil was not the magic formula they hoped it would be. It fell out of favor with even the most hopeful physicians.

Doctors had complete authority and power over what was done to their patients' bodies, how they spent their days, what they ate, whom they could see, and a constant barrage of unpleasantness. But surrender to these indignities meant getting something else, and next to being discharged, it was what the patients hoped for most.

They called it an "up."

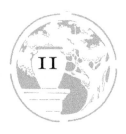

YOUR GREATEST WISH
WILL BE GRANTED

UPS WERE PRIVILEGES, rewards, and barometers. Only patients who had weeks of low temps, negative sputum, and significant weight gain got ups. Ups were the opposite of rest, and when a woman was told she could be up for a few hours a day, she mentally started packing for home.

An up could be anything: a walk to the outdoor balconies with a book on a nice day, a meal in the dining room, a short car ride into Fairfax to do a little shopping, or even a trip into San Francisco for a stylish new haircut. These were tests, to see if movement and a pretense at real life would bring on the old symptoms. Doctors observed patients for a long time before pronouncing them ready to leave, and ups were as much a diagnostic tool as the X-ray.

By the late 1920s, the doctor who had the final say on when patients could get up, walk around, or go home was Philip King Brown's son Cabot.

He had followed family tradition to enter medicine, and his youth was spent at good San Francisco schools and in the family's philanthropic activities, which were not always fun for a kid. When he was eight years old, he and his older brother, Hillyer, danced minuets dressed like eighteenth-century courtiers at a benefit for the Armitage Orphanage in nearby San Mateo. Their female partners were from equally philanthropic and wealthy families.

Like his father, Cabot Brown went to Harvard, but he seems to have taken after his precocious and brilliant grandmother Dr. Charlotte Brown: he enrolled in 1917 when he was just fifteen. The following year he enlisted in the infantry and served in the Students' Army Training Corps in Plattsburg, New York, though the war ended before he saw action overseas. He completed his BA in 1921 and then entered Harvard's medical school.

A few years into his training, Cabot decided to take a breather from college. He had entered Harvard when he was just a teenager and wanted some time to enjoy his youth, so he spent a year traveling the world. In China he met a vivacious American woman named Margaret Keeley, known as Peggy, who was also on a grand tour. The two kept in touch after his return to Harvard and her return home to Chicago, and they were married in 1926, the year he received his MD.

His proud father gave him some advice when he came back to San Francisco to start his career. He had been offered the opportunity to intern at Stanford, but Philip Brown suggested that Cabot instead spend three mornings a week at Southern Pacific Hospital, where Philip was a visiting physician. This would give Cabot valuable experience with many kinds of illness and injuries, and would also allow him to open his own practice. He soon had an office next door to his father on Hyde Street near St. Francis Hospital.

Cabot soon decided to focus on chest diseases, and in 1933 he realized he needed some additional training. A medical school friend who ran a tuberculosis hospital in Connecticut offered Cabot a crash course in thoracic surgery, as well as other treatments, which would give him the knowledge of a year's residency in three intense months. He had a wife and two small children at home, so this was the best solution for everyone.[1]

Patients remembered Philip King Brown as a warm and sympathetic doctor, despite a natural reserve. But Cabot Brown was another story. He had an energetic, optimistic personality and a sense of humor, and as he bounded around the wards like a friendly dog, his cheeriness was a balm for frightened patients. In 1927 he worked his magic on a terrified housewife from Sonoma: Lois Downey.

~

On a cold November day, Lois and Harvey Downey drove their car off a San Francisco Bay ferry and onto downtown streets toward Dr. Philip King Brown's office. Once inside, they huddled together on chairs in his waiting room until a nurse called Lois's name. After she sat alone in the examining room for a few minutes, Dr. Brown walked in with a soft smile. He talked to her, listened to her lungs, and looked at her X-rays and medical records. He was friendly and seemed sympathetic. He then told her she could get dressed and went back into the waiting room, where he had a quick and uncomfortable conversation with Harvey.

Lois had advanced-stage tuberculosis, he said, which meant that a sanatorium rest cure would probably not make her well. Dr. Brown sent women to Arequipa only if they were in the early stages of TB because they had the best hope for being cured. Heartsick, Harvey asked how long his wife had. Probably just three months, Dr. Brown told him, confirming what their own physician had said. Harvey then thought for a moment and asked the doctor if he would make an exception. Would he take Lois for three months to see if she would improve? If she didn't make any progress, he would take her home to die.

Philip King Brown thought for a moment and then agreed. He had made the rare exception to his policy in the past in extraordinary circumstances, and since he had a few available beds at the moment, he thought giving Lois even a slight chance for recovery was better than none. He told the anxious Harvey that Lois could stay at Arequipa for ninety days and they would reevaluate her condition then. When Lois joined them, both men told her she would indeed go to the sanatorium that very day, and then Dr. Brown told her what to expect.

"You won't see a lot of sickly, pale, anemic looking people at Arequipa, because that's not what they are," he said. "They've all got plenty of weight on them and they've got rosy cheeks and they're happy, and it's not going to be what you think." This didn't make sense to her, but she took him at his word, too distracted to really listen.

Harvey and Lois drove off the return ferry and back into Marin County, heading west on the county road that led directly to Arequipa's stone entry gates, one of Henry Bothin's gifts to the sanatorium. Motoring up the hill to the building, Lois had a passing thought about the beauty of the tree-filled grounds, but she was too scared and cold to pay attention. Her spirits did not improve when she walked into the cavernous sanatorium and found that it wasn't much warmer than it was outside. She said a quick and awful good-bye to her husband as an efficient nurse took her arm and led her away. She was put into her pajamas, her other things were unpacked, and she was bundled into a bed. Then the tears came and she turned over to keep them quiet, wondering if she would ever leave this chilly, gloomy place.

When my grandmother Lois Downey entered Arequipa that 1927 winter day, she was the beneficiary of more than fifteen years of trial, error, staff changes, and medical improvements. Her experience at Arequipa was everything Dr. Philip King Brown hoped for, and each day of the fourteen months she would lie in her bed was the sanatorium rest cure in action.

Fifty years after leaving Arequipa, Lois remembered every detail of her stay. Food was one of the sharpest memories—not for its taste but because of how fast she put weight back on. She gained twenty-six pounds in three months, and she knew the reason why: "I went up like a balloon . . . you get a lot of starchy food. You had puddings, you had potatoes and had things that weren't exactly good for anybody that wanted to be on a diet, but it was very plain food, as I remember it. But apparently nourishing. It certainly nourished me."

Those pounds kept her at Arequipa. Her three-month probation period ended in February 1928. The doctors quietly conferred, and Philip King Brown called Harvey to say that Lois was responding to treatment and could stay at Arequipa until she was symptom-free. She had become one of the rosy-cheeked brigade, and it wasn't until decades later that her husband told her about the deal he had made with Dr. Brown.

Lois became a candidate for pneumothorax after her probation was over. Her overall condition was better, but one day she had a small hemorrhage, and the doctors decided that it was time to intervene. The problem was her left lung, which had a hole the size of a doorknob. One morning a nurse came for Lois and helped her wobble to the treatment room and lie down for her first pneumo. She never forgot it:

> They had a little machine with a long hollow needle that was connected to this machine with a hose, and it was pumping air, and the needle would be inserted between the ribs. They started on the back first and then when the air would go in around the lung itself and in the pleura of the lung, and it would collapse the lung, and they told me that it would look like a piece of liver rather than a lung. Some of the patients could hold that air for weeks, and [with] others, it would seep out somehow or other. I had to have it every week for quite some time, and then I got to the point where I could hold it a little bit longer. For some reason or another, everyone wasn't the same.
>
> That's what it did. It collapsed the lung, and they also used the same needle when I got fluid on the lung, and [they] drew the fluid out, and it was the most beautiful green that you would ever see in your life, just a deep emerald green. I looked at it, because you were always conscious, you weren't anesthetized or anything going through this, and I said to the doctor, what a beautiful color, and he said, "Yes, that's pure poison."

That lovely green fluid was infected pus from around her lung, called purulent exudate, or empyema. Because it was in the pleural cavity, she couldn't "cough it out" or otherwise expel it. So, the pneumo treatment was as much for removing contagion as it was collapsing the compromised, tubercular lung itself.

While she generally got an X-ray about once a month, she and the other patients lined up for the fluoroscope more often, sometimes weekly. The nurses would bring a group of women to the dark room reserved for the machine and sit them down in a row.

"When it came our turn we'd get up, and the nurse would be there and take us by the arm and see that we get over there without falling down and stand us up there," Lois remembered. And the procedure itself was more energetic than an X-ray: "They would stand you up in front of the light, this flat plate that was hanging from the ceiling, and they would just move it back and forth, push it this way, push it that way, and it could get a very good picture of the lung."

Lois and another young woman were a challenge for the technicians: "We were the same size and had the same problem apparently, because they couldn't tell us apart until we told them who we were. They told us to give our name when we stepped up there because they knew the rest of them as well as they knew their face, by looking at their lungs, but the trouble was that we were too much alike, so we just gave our names."

Arequipa's doctors and nurses seem to have done a good job explaining why they were doing these mysterious procedures. "They went very much by that, much better than an X-ray because it was live, you were there, your heart was beating and everything. It was very good, very easy, I guess, for them."

And Lois also knew about the surgeries, because women in her ward had disappeared to hospitals and then returned, telling horror stories of their procedures: "They also had another one called phrenectomy. They cut a little muscle in the neck, and that would bring the lung up. Usually that was done when you had trouble in the lower lobe, and that would collapse just the lower lobe. Of course, there was the thoracoplasty, which was the worst one of all, where they take out a piece of your rib and dismantle your lung completely."

Despite her less-than-hopeful diagnosis, Arequipa's routine was slowly making Lois well, although she wasn't allowed to play bridge because her temperature always went up after a few rubbers. But death was on her mind anyway. "After the first week, I knew by that time I was there to stay until I got well or stepped off the end," she recalled. It didn't help that one young woman did die when she was at Arequipa:

She put up such a fight. She never moved either. She did everything they told her to do, but she had lost a brother and a sister and most of her family from tuberculosis, and it was just one of those things. She just wasn't supposed to get well. She had been in there for months, and she would just lie so still and [was] a nice sweet young woman. They finally took her up to the nurses' quarters because she was too bad.... We knew she died there, but none of us could prove it. That's what was said. We weren't supposed to hear about things like that.

Lois loved the nurses, though she couldn't recall all their names:

We had one young one there. I don't know if I still have a picture of her or not. She was awfully nice—friendly and full of pep and pleasant. All the rest of them were gray-haired women, and some of them were almost too old. There was Mrs. Ford, and she was awfully nice, but she shouldn't have been working. She was getting pretty old. There were a lot of steps for them to take from one ward to the other and all through that great big building.

Elizabeth MacMillan was a special favorite:

Miss MacMillan . . . came down in our ward one day and was telling us she was up in the upper ward, and there was a girl standing up by the table and she was just fiddling around, not doing anything. So Miss MacMillan didn't say anything to her at all, and she walked down through the ward to see if there was anything she needed to do and came back, and this girl said, "I'm standing up." Miss MacMillan said, "I see you are." And she said, "Why don't you tell me to go to bed?" And Miss Macmillan said, "I told her I thought she knew enough to without being told."

Lois had great respect for the formidable Ethel Steeves. Even though she was the superintendent, she "came right down and made beds with the rest of them, and they all worked just the same. She was strict and would say something to you if you weren't doing the right thing." Lois never forgot one particular sheet-changing day.

She was sitting in the chair near her bed while Steeves wrestled with her bed linens. Lois was still weak and tired, and she sat in the chair unmoving, staring at the screened wall, not chattering like her ward mates were. As Steeves finished tucking the blankets in place, she walked over to Lois, leaned over, kissed her on the forehead, and walked briskly away.

Lois said that the doctors and nurses were all a special type of person: "I think it was probably important that they were pleasant and friendly to the patients and would greet us with a smile, that sort of thing. I can't say that there was one of them that I ever felt made me unhappy. I was pleased to see them all."

~

Optimistic and socially inclined, Lois soon got over her initial fear and home-sickness, and then tried to blend in and make friends. Arequipa had a small library where all the donated books were kept, and the ambulatory girls would help the bed patients choose titles they were interested in. Lois chose a book on palmistry one day and read it in between meals and naps over the next few days. Once she finished it, her neighbors started asking her to read their palms. She had a knack for the theatrical and made every reading very dramatic, which she thought was amusing, especially when the women believed everything she said.

Her reputation got around to the other wards. A fellow patient asked Lois to read her mother's palm one afternoon when she came by to visit. Lois took the woman's hand and in a gypsy-like voice said, "I see an accident." The woman gasped, "Oh, my God, not another one!" She had almost been killed in a car accident once, so Lois hastily replied, "Oh, it's already passed!" She was more careful after that and foresaw only love and success from then on.

Not everyone could end up as friends, but most women tried and seemed to understand that their unusual living situation demanded a different way of looking at life. Lois had her emotions "very much under control," as she put it. "We were all there for the same thing, and I think that's why we all got along well together."

This attitude also extended to the nonwhite patients. An Asian American in Lois's ward was the only woman of color at Arequipa the entire time she was there, but Lois didn't think this was because of discrimination. "I can't picture them being that discriminating, when someone was ill," she said. "To take me when I was as bad as I was—they really didn't have to take me at all, and I just feel that if there had been someone that had needed it, no matter what their race was, they would have taken them. I would hope that was the way it was." She didn't say if any of the other patients had trouble sharing a close space with the "Chinese girl," but it's very likely that not everyone was happy about her being there. Anyone who did feel this way had to keep her thoughts to herself.

Clashes erupted, of course. Sometimes, all the women could do was tolerate one another. But other times the group had to exert its will on the more disruptive individuals.

Lois remembered one woman whose abrasive personality and personal habits (mostly having to do with the way she used dental floss) drove everyone crazy and whose bed was just two over from hers. One day the unpleasant patient was in the bathroom when her lunch tray was delivered, so Lois quietly slipped from under the covers and over to the other woman's bed.

She lifted the cover off the food plate and found the piece of chocolate candy that was their treat for the day. In her hand was a butter knife and the pepper shaker from her own tray. She quickly sliced off the bottom of the candy, filled the inside with as much pepper as she could, put the bottom back on, and smoothed over the break. She scooted back to her bed and a few minutes later the woman returned from the bathroom. Everyone ate their lunch but kept their eyes casually trained on her every move.

After the victim finished her meal, she reached for her candy, took a bite, and then made a face as her cheeks turned red and she began to cough. She headed for the bathroom more quickly than the TB glide allowed, and when she came back, her ward mates were innocently chatting with one another. No one ever said a thing about the incident, but even though the patient continued to be irritating, Lois and her cronies felt they had done something for the collective peace of their ward.

Peace descended on most Sundays. A priest came by once a month to hear confessions from the Catholic patients, and the doctor's private office was turned into a makeshift confessional. Two of Lois's favorite ward mates were young sisters whose father was a police officer in San Francisco. She called them "the Irish girls," and Helen was the more high-spirited of the two. One Sunday morning after seeing the priest, Helen sauntered back to the ward, stood in the doorway, and said, "You sons of bitches. I can do anything I want to for the next month. I've just been to confession!"

Holidays were difficult for the patients, and the staff did what they could to ease the pain of being away from family and friends. Even though husbands, children, and parents were allowed to visit during regular hours throughout the year, not everyone could make the trip. Until the Golden Gate Bridge was completed in 1937, anyone coming from across the bay still had to take the ferry to Marin County, which didn't always operate in bad weather. The trains out to Fairfax could be temperamental too. So not everyone had the comfort of familiar faces on December 25.

Christmas of 1927 came just a month after Lois entered Arequipa, and she was one of the lucky ones. Her husband and son were able to come and see her, taking the easy drive south from Sonoma. To help make the season festive, the nurses and other staff members put up a tree in the living room, and the patients made little gifts for one another using craft supplies that benefactors donated just for that purpose. They hung them on the tree, and everyone had a present on Christmas morning. They did the same during Lois's second holiday season, of 1928. A year into her cure she was doing well and the sanatorium routine was second nature, but she never got used to watching her son grow up in only sporadic viewings on visiting days or holidays.

Like the other patients, Lois had to put up with all kinds of weather in her big, screened ward. In the California summers, which in July and August could approach one hundred degrees, Arequipa's little valley stayed cooler. The winter fog that counties near San Francisco are famous for also made a frequent appearance, and not just outside. Lois recalled those days for their clamminess, but also for where the fog went: "There would be days when the fog would drift along through the hills, and we were just high enough that it would just drift into the ward there. It didn't happen very often, but it was quite interesting to us when it did happen because you could look down at the other end of the ward and it would be fog all the way along."

Of all the staff she saw each day, Lois remembered Dr. Cabot Brown with the greatest affection. "Oh, he was just a great big good-natured kid. I just loved him. He was so nice, a great big smile on his face. He looked like a football player—he was so tall and so big. He would just come in like a big brother. [He] asked how I was and always seemed to be so pleased that I was getting along fine."

Cabot Brown looked after his patients well beyond their TB diagnosis. In the fall of 1928 smallpox broke out in nearby Oakland and Berkeley, and Cabot decided to vaccinate all the women at Arequipa. He took this on himself and went down the ward, bed by bed, giving the vaccine by scratching the surface of the skin of every patient. When he got to Lois, he said, "I think I'll do two, just to be sure." She always chuckled about what happened next: "Well, both of them took. I had the sorest arm—swollen, sore, and you wouldn't believe the scar I had there. Two scars—one right alongside the other, about an inch long. I remember about the time I was getting ready to leave there, he was examining me and he says, 'When are you going to sue me?'"

Lois cared what Cabot Brown thought of her, and she tried hard to take his advice and be a good patient. After she had the hemorrhage a few months into her stay, Cabot told her he was disappointed because up until then she had been his star patient. Even the other women remarked on how well she had been doing. "They used to tell me themselves that so-and-so was not near as bad as I was when they came in. I was noted for never moving—just lie there without ever moving at all. When I got to feeling too homesick, I got to counting knot-holes in the ceiling."

Cabot Brown held Lois up as an example to other patients who couldn't be restful. They would get out of bed to wander over to a table to get a magazine when they had no up privileges, or if they were allowed to move around, they would zoom from one place to the other instead of gliding. If a patient wasn't following the rules, Cabot's sunny face would turn very stern and a forthright lecture would follow, with Lois as its frequent object lesson. "You're not getting well as fast as Mrs. Downey, and you aren't near as bad as she was," he sometimes told them.

But even after getting regular pneumothorax treatments, gaining weight, and suffering no more relapses, Lois was never offered an up. She watched other women ask for time out of bed or even ask when they were going home. But as they were turned down or, even worse, relapsed instead of improving, she decided to just keep her mouth shut, follow the rules, and wait for the doctors to tell her she was ready.

By the beginning of 1929, fourteen months into her stay, Lois began to have recurring dreams of sparkling clear waters, blue horizons, sunshine, and, occasionally, snow. One of her ward mates was very interested in dreams and would interpret them for the other patients. When Lois told her about the snow-filled ones, she said, "If you dream about snow, your greatest wish will be granted."

One day in late January 1929, Cabot Brown and the nurses were talking near Lois's bed about a woman who desperately needed to come to Arequipa, but because all the beds were filled there wasn't any room for her. Without thinking, Lois spoke up: "Why don't you give her my bed?" Cabot turned to Lois and said, "Do you want to go home?" She replied that she did, very much, as long as she was well enough. He then said, "You could have gone home before this, but we didn't think you wanted to."

Startled, Lois assured him she was more than ready, so over the next month they let her spend a little bit of time every day on her feet, eating in the dining room, going to the bathroom on her own, sitting on the balcony, and other delightful activities. The doctors took more X-rays and then Cabot Brown sat her down to tell her she could leave, but she needed to hear a few things first. He was more serious than she had ever seen him: "He told me the doctors had had a meeting . . . but they didn't know how I was going to make out emotionally because they felt I had emotional problems that had brought this on. So they felt that if my problems weren't cleared up by the time I went home, that I'd be back there again."

Lois knew what he meant. She had always clashed with her opinionated mother-in-law, a situation made worse because they lived next door to each other. She wanted to raise her son her own way, but the other Mrs. Downey didn't agree with her methods and did not hesitate to let her know about it. The two women battled almost constantly, with little Harvey Jr. in the middle. Cabot Brown said these confrontations were dangerous to someone trying to recover from TB. Lois knew that she would have to make peace with her mother-in-law for her own sake, as much as for her son's. She'd learned a lot at Arequipa and told Dr. Brown so.

February gives northern Californians a preview of spring to come. The heavy rains of January cease, and warm temperatures coax the buds of flowering trees to open. Daffodils, jonquils, and other bulbs practically jump out of the soil. It's a lovely breather between what can be an icy start to the year and the coming winds and returning rains of March. On a bright afternoon around Valentine's Day, Lois walked out of the French doors and onto the tiled patio, accompanied by a nurse carrying a Brownie camera. Wearing a flowered kimono and embroidered slippers, Lois smoothed her short, dark hair and beamed as the nurse took her picture. The nurse sent the film away for developing, and Lois was able to put the snapshot into her purse a few days later.

Near the end of the month, she packed her suitcase, wearing a new dress her husband had brought her, which was three sizes larger than she was used to. Nearly thirty pounds heavier now, she couldn't fit into the dress she'd worn on that cold November admission day so long before. She then walked around the building, saying good-bye to the women who for more than a year had shared her ward, her fears, and the chairs in the treatment room. A few faces were new, but even they had become important to her. She knew how they felt. She thanked the nurses and had also given Cabot Brown a tearful thank-you at their final meeting.

Arequipa's up patients lingered on the balconies from late morning to early afternoon on these soft early spring days. A few minutes after lunch was over, they saw a car drive through the stone gates and up the long driveway. It stopped near the main building, and tall, lanky Harvey Downey got out of the car and waited. Watching from Arequipa's doorway, Lois saw him and then turned to gather up her suitcase, purse, and hat. She made a quick but smooth dash back into her ward and waved with unashamed tears in her eyes to the women on chairs and in beds, who were nearly all as tearful. Then she turned, walked out the door, and walked into the sun.[2]

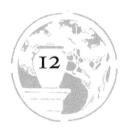

12

A WORLD WITHIN A WORLD

WHEN WOMEN WERE DISCHARGED FROM AREQUIPA, their empty beds looked strange to those who were left behind. But no one really grieved, because they all hoped for their own day of departure. Besides, new patients arrived and routines took over, in medical treatment and in opportunities for entertainment and diversion. This continued to be very important, both to Dr. Brown and to his patients. So in 1930, after a hiatus of nearly a decade, the latest crop of Arequipa patients decided to put another magazine together. They called it *The Mountaineer*. *Hi-Life* had survived until the end of 1922, and there was a long dormant period before *The Mountaineer* came off the presses. Once under way, it took a very different tone from its predecessors. The front page of each issue contained a short, instructive essay about taking the TB cure, either written by one of the patients or a well-known doctor or reprinted from a medical journal.

The September 15, 1931, issue, for example, started off with an article titled "What Are We Taught At Arequipa?" The writer was a patient who had absorbed Philip King Brown's credo of "sanatorium as school," as well as the corollary that each patient was responsible for her own cure by obeying the rules and by cultivating the proper attitude of optimism. "If by good fortune one has had the intelligence to avail herself of Arequipa's teachings, its aim has been attained," wrote the anonymous essayist. "But if not there should be no reflection on the institution . . . rather the limitations of the individual," she concluded.[1]

After this instructional beginning, the rest of the issue contained news about current and former patients, and light humor reminiscent of *Hi-Life*. There were fewer articles about hijinks, though, and more mentions of board members' visits and the donations they made. In the early 1930s, *The Mountaineer* was also mailed to former patients, and many of them wrote thank-you notes, glad to be kept informed about the progress of the friends they had made during their time there. *The Mountaineer* also printed articles about staff members, and soon the reporters had new ones to talk about.

Ethel Steeves left Arequipa sometime in 1929, and after a few months' searching, the board of directors found Eva Gregg, who took over as superintendent in January 1930. Born in Michigan in 1886, she graduated from the Butterworth Hospital School for Nurses in Grand Rapids and took a job at the hospital. Three years later she was nursing at the Lockwood Hospital and Deaconess' Home in Petoskey, Michigan. Then she upended her life.

A devout member of the Methodist Episcopal Church, she decided to add missionary to her résumé and in 1912 she sailed to Shanghai from San Francisco on the SS *Manchuria*, notable for being one of the first transpacific ships to carry cows so that passengers could have fresh milk. She then began work as a nurse at the church's mission in Tientsin, China, a port city in the northeastern part of the country. She also worked at the Isabella Fisher Hospital there, supervised nurses at foreign hospitals in Tientsin and in Beijing (then called Peking), and started up a nurse training school in Tientsin. In 1914 she supervised workers in charge of constructing a new building for the Isabella Fisher Hospital. She was praised by one of the doctors for her work as "building inspector" and for her compassion for patients' health: "Their confidence in her ability was so great that they called her 'doctor' and begged for medicine and for dressing for their wounds. For three months, in sunshine and rain, she continued, until we secured the services of an American builder."

Between 1912 and 1928, Eva Gregg made multiple trips between China and the United States, coming home to raise funds for the mission and, in 1922, for famine relief. That year she sailed via Seattle and gave an interview to journalists about her work. "There is so much to be done in China, and the number of nurses is so inadequate," she said. "A vast amount of good is being done in teaching the Chinese better sanitation in their homes; but the big need is for nurses to attend the sick."

She came home for good in 1927 and lived with her father for a while in Bozeman, Montana. A year later she moved west to Oakland, California, working as the assistant superintendent of nurses at the city's Highland Hospital School of Nursing. She then crossed paths with Philip King Brown. He asked her to succeed Ethel Steeves as superintendent, and she accepted, moving to the cottage on the grounds reserved for the woman in charge.

The patients took to Gregg right away. They even dedicated a poem to her on the cover of the September 15, 1931, issue of the *Mountaineer*. Titled "Because of You," it was written by a patient with the initials V. M.:

You stood beside my bed
  and smiled.
Gave encouragement
  the while
I looked about the San
  and knew
That it is just like home
  because of you.

Eva Gregg never forgot China, and she brought the country and its needs into her new life at Arequipa. The very month she started as superintendent, she gave a talk about her missionary work to the San Rafael Improvement Club. In February 1932 she spoke about her time in China to members of a local Congregational church. A few months later she hosted naval commander Lyman Swenson and his wife for lunch at Arequipa and introduced them as people she had known in Shanghai.

She knew how important it was to have pleasant surroundings at a hospital. Calling on her previous experience as a "building inspector," Gregg pushed through another renovation project at Arequipa in the fall of 1932. The sanatorium had not been repainted since 1919, and painting was well overdue. The walls were painted in tones of yellow and pale green, chairs were recovered with brightly colored flowered fabric, and potted ferns were placed throughout the public areas.

Many Arequipa patients wrote letters to the board of directors about how kind and thoughtful Superintendent Gregg was, even while they were still in bed taking the cure. One correspondent was a twenty-five-year-old stenographer from Oakland who was married and on the brink of divorce. She entered the sanatorium in January 1932 after a breakdown caused by her husband's cruelty and intemperance (hence the pending divorce). She wrote her letter a few weeks after she was admitted, saying she was pleased with Arequipa and knew she would be contented: "The girls have been so nice to me and made me feel right at home, also Miss Gregg and the nurses. I know I am going to get well quickly in these pleasant surroundings."

She ended her letter with a PS: "Please do not give information to anyone, even should members of my family inquire, without my written consent." This likely meant her husband. She needn't have worried; the staff was very strict about patient confidentiality.[2]

Eva Gregg worked closely with Dr. Ethel Owen, who had come back to Arequipa in early 1925 after her trip to Europe. Dr. Owen was fast becoming a tuberculosis expert. Speaking to a meeting of the California Tuberculosis Association in San Jose in December 1928, she warned about the dangers of the "boyish figure" fad among young women (flappers), whose TB rates had been rising even as rates fell among young men.

In May 1930 a reporter interviewed Dr. Owen about her work with San Francisco's Community Chest, a fund-raising organization founded in Ohio in 1913 that funneled its donations to a variety of charities. Nearly every major city had a Community Chest (which explains its appearance in the Monopoly board game), and San Francisco's branch paid the fees for many Arequipa patients over the years.

In this interview, Dr. Owen condemned strict diets and a flapper lifestyle as the reason for the continued rise in TB among women between fifteen and thirty-five. She also thought sunbathing was bad for the lungs, with the exception of heliotherapy—a sunbathing treatment of glandular and bone tuberculosis.

Ethel Owen took on another job in 1930: Arequipa's medical director. Philip King Brown had slowly backed away from those duties as he got older, because the sanatorium's routine had long been in place and Cabot was now walking the wards. He was confident in his choice of successor, as Dr. Owen's expertise in TB made her the perfect candidate. She was also affiliated with the San Francisco Board of Health and was making public health another personal mission. She was a member of the city's Business and Professional Women's Club and gave a talk on TB prevention to club members in August 1930.

Whether as attending physician or administrator, she earned the deep affection of Arequipa's patients. The August 15, 1931, issue of *The Mountaineer* included a poem written by V. M., titled "Your Smile" and dedicated to Dr. Owen.

> As the dew-drop helps the thirsty rose,
> As night lulls day to sweet repose,
> So your smile helps our hungry souls.
> As the sunrise beautifies the dawn,
> As a mirrored lake reflects the swan,
> So your smile helps our days along.
> As a friend that's always near at hand,
> So with eyes that cheer but not command,
> Your smile helps this Arequipa band.

Dr. Owen and Dr. Adelaide Brown had become good friends, despite a twenty-two-year gap in their ages. They probably met through their mutual interests and work at Stanford. Adelaide had been appointed a lecturer in child hygiene at the university in 1920 and would no doubt have come into contact with Dr. Owen when she was the women students' medical adviser. In the spring of 1931 the two women took a house together in San Anselmo for the summer, which made Owen's commute to Arequipa much shorter. They returned to San Francisco in the fall and then faced a crisis.

On September 28 Ethel Owen underwent emergency surgery for a bowel obstruction and was in grave danger for a couple of weeks. By mid-October she was recuperating at Adelaide Brown's home, near where her brother Philip and his wife, Helen, still lived, in the house they had built after the 1906 earthquake and fire. (Philip and Adelaide's father, Henry Brown, who had lived with Adelaide since Charlotte's death in 1904, had passed away in 1930.) Ethel Owen was well enough to go out to Arequipa with Adelaide a week before Halloween to judge the all-sanatorium costume contest. The October 26 issue of *The Mountaineer*, which reported on the contest, had a special front page: "This issue of The Mountaineer is affectionately dedicated to the speedy recovery of our dear Dr. Ethel D. Owen."

Dr. Owen made a point to speak publicly about TB prevention whenever she could. In 1933 she addressed the California Tuberculosis Society's convention in San Diego: "Of paramount importance is the need of the public to understand the four fundamental truths in controlling tuberculosis, namely: A case of tuberculosis comes from another case of tuberculosis; tuberculosis is preventable; tuberculosis is never hereditary, and the best results in treatment of tuberculosis come from cases diagnosed early."[3]

She also followed the medical fortunes of many of the patients she treated at Arequipa. In 1932 a twenty-eight-year-old woman entered the sanatorium after being referred by Isabel Dibblee, Philip King Brown's benefactor from Marin County. She was a former telephone operator now working as a hairdresser, whose husband had deserted her when she got pregnant. A few years after her child was born, she collapsed with bronchiectasis, a disease that inflames the bronchi of the lungs and that can become cystic fibrosis. She spent a little over three months at Arequipa but couldn't stay any longer because she couldn't pay for both her treatment and whatever solution she had found for child care. She had improved though. Dr. Owen was glad about that, and she wrote to the woman regularly to make sure she kept on seeing her own doctor. In a letter to Dr. Owen, the former patient told her, "I certainly appreciate what Arequipa has done for me."

Ethel Owen also followed up with a patient whose personal story seemed to come right out of a tearjerker. She was a divorced housewife of thirty-two, whose father had died of TB and whose sister was also afflicted, though taking the rest cure at home. She found out she had first-stage TB and pleuritis and entered Arequipa in January 1932. She had some money from her divorce settlement and a small legacy from her grandparents, and the San Francisco Tuberculosis Association made up the deficit in her fees out of a special fund that helped desperately ill and poor people get sanatorium care.

The patient had had two legal abortions because of her health and was both a smoker and a drinker—habits she had to give up when she was in the sanatorium. Her mother lived out of town, and the woman did not want her to know she had tuberculosis, so her sister helped out with her children's care, despite her own tubercular condition.

The patient was very emotional and nervous. She cried a lot and managed to stay at Arequipa for only three months, partly because of costs and partly because she couldn't handle the routine. After she was discharged, she wrote to Dr. Owen, complaining about the doctor she was seeing: "I want to thank you for your patience with me—you've had a bad patient to deal with—I sometimes wonder if I'm not mentally a wreck—all I can do lately is cry! & cry! I can understand why so many TBs take their own lives if it affects them mentally, as it seems to have me."

Dr. Owen wrote back, urging her to rest and to go to the San Francisco Polyclinic if she could, to get additional advice and care. She also told her to "try in every way to overcome your emotional reaction. Tears are not very useful in the cure of TB."[4]

⁓

There may have been more tears in the wards in the months after the 1929 stock market crash and the domino effect of job losses that followed. The Depression jolted the husbands and other family members at home who paid for their women's care at Arequipa. But if the patients were concerned about the country's financial condition, the subject didn't find its way into the pages of *The Mountaineer*. The opening essay of the October 25, 1931, issue makes clear that this was deliberate:

We are living temporarily in a world within a world, a world apart. Did you ever think of it that way? Our contacts with the outside are seldom direct ones and for that reason cannot be of much interest or help to us. Our interests must be here, where we are, and since our world is a small one, they must be less exclusively personal. It is easy to be self-centered in that other world—easy but not wise; in our life it is difficult and so unwise as to be unallowed. Here, even so vague a thing as one's mental attitude can affect, seriously affect, the happiness of others. Perhaps happiness is an ill-chosen word: let us say rather well-being.[5]

Elsie Krafft, who was still the resident social worker, continued to document the professions of the women admitted to Arequipa, and as the Depression got under way, the balance between working patients and housewives remained. Stenographers, telephone operators, and students were among the most common admissions after the housewives.

Eva Gregg decided to leave Arequipa in November 1934 to work in an unnamed city hospital near San Francisco. Local newspapers covered her departure, describing her as a well-liked member of the sanatorium staff. A nurse named Marybeth Farnsworth took over as temporary superintendent. She was a California native who got her nursing degree at Highland Hospital nursing school in Oakland in 1930 and then worked at the hospital until she took the job at Arequipa. She was in place just a few months. Then, in early 1935, Emma Applegren came on board.[6]

Like Dr. Ethel Owen and Philip King Brown himself, Applegren had gone to France during World War I. Michigan-born in 1891, she got her nursing degree in 1914 at the Passavant Memorial Hospital School of Nursing, which was affiliated with Northwestern University in Chicago.

In 1917 she signed up with the Red Cross to serve as a nurse overseas and joined Northwestern's Base Hospital 12. The group of doctors and nurses left Chicago on May 16, and their ship, the SS *Mongolia*, left New York on May 19, carrying more than four hundred medical volunteers from all over the country. One day out, during a test of the ship's guns, a shell exploded as it hit the water, scattering shrapnel onto the deck, killing two nurses and wounding another. Rather than bury the women at sea, the ship's captain turned back to return the bodies to their families. The *Mongolia* sailed again for Europe on May 22.

After spending time in England, the Northwestern unit set up at a general hospital in Dannes-Camiers, in the north of France near the English Channel.

Emma Applegren and the other volunteers stayed there until April 1919. Within a year after her return to the States, Applegren was working as a public health nurse in Hillsdale, Michigan. She taught classes in infant care and went house to house as a community nurse for the next six years, traveling more than fifty thousand miles in her car to attend to her work and her patients.

She then heard about a position at the city hospital in San Jose, California, and moved there in August 1926. She liked California, and in 1930 she became the nursing supervisor at Sutter Hospital in Sacramento. She was then either recruited for or heard about the Superintendent position at Arequipa. Like her predecessors, she showed up in the latest iteration of the sanatorium's magazine.[7]

The patients took a vote to change *The Mountaineer*'s title in 1935. The new name was *Quipa-Tab*. One of its early editors had established a little store at the sanatorium, where patients could buy niceties such as thimbles, thread, and magazines. The profits were so great that sanatorium volunteers could buy flowers and gifts for the patients rather than relying solely on donations to buy them. And they used some of the extra money to get *Quipa-Tab* professionally printed. Someone managed to get local businesses to take out ads to help cover some of the expenses too. Advertisers include the Marin County Milk Company in San Rafael.

Quipa-Tab was more literary than its original incarnation. It followed the instructional bent of previous years but also kept up with the long-standing tradition of in-house humor. The want ads were a popular regular feature:

For Winona U.—An extra 8 hours a day so she can do more sketching.
For Virginia C.—Someone to do her talking for her so she can take a
     good cure.
For Alice E.—More books.
For Miss Applegren—1 pair of pruning shears (shh, it's supposed to be
     a secret, but did you know, girls, that she likes to go around and
     accidentally snip off flowers?).[8]

Emma Applegren also brought something to her job that was very different from her predecessors: two dogs, cairn terriers named Ladye Buffe Craig and Ladye Heather Lumsden, who were allowed to come into the wards now and then. The best days were those when consulting physician Dr. Leo Eloesser visited, because he also brought along a dog, a dachshund named Adolph. He apparently ignored the two females, which delighted a writer for *Quipa-Tab* so much that she had to write something up for the magazine: "Languishing looks of entreaty are of no avail and so fascinating Buffe and piquant Heather have their heads together trying to find out their lack of appeal."⁹

Applegren also worked with civic and charitable institutions to help patients pay for treatment at Arequipa. The number of women who needed help of all kinds increased during the Depression years. In August 1931, the Lions Club in the nearby towns of San Rafael and San Anselmo heard that the movie projector at Arequipa worked only with silent films. "Talkies" had firmly supplanted the silents, and the Lions felt that the patients deserved to see the most up-to-date movies. Club members held luncheons at Arequipa and planned fund-raisers, where money for a sound projector was raised in record time.

The Community Chest continued to cover the costs for poorer patients, and the organization used their personal stories in annual appeals for funds. In February 1931 the *San Francisco Chronicle* published the story of a Mrs. S.

Her husband had died, and Mrs. S. worked hard to support herself and her baby. She was troubled by a strange pain in her wrist, so she went to a clinic at the University of California hospital in San Francisco and found out she had tuberculosis. She appealed to the Community Chest for help, and not only was she admitted to Arequipa, but the Infant Shelter took care of her baby. (This was a charity that Arequipa benefactor Mary Holton supported for decades.) Mrs. S. spent a few months at Arequipa, where "quiet and nourishing food arrested the disease and now Mrs. S. is back at work again." The article ended with the lesson the Community Chest hoped that readers would remember: Mrs. S. "carefully follows the regime prescribed for her by the social worker from Arequipa." The Community Chest published stories about Arequipa almost yearly throughout the 1930s.

Some New Deal programs within California also helped the sanatorium's patients, though in a different way. In 1933 the State Emergency Relief Administration (SERA) was created to distribute state and federal funds to people affected by the Depression. In January 1935 California had a SERA orchestra. Its musicians played a concert at Arequipa and at the county's poor farm.¹⁰

In September 1936 another orchestra, this one funded by the federal Works Progress Administration, played at Arequipa's twenty-fifth anniversary party. Nearly one hundred former patients, members of the press, and dignitaries converged on the sanatorium and listened to Philip King Brown relate its history and its successes before the festivities began.

In the quarter century since Arequipa was founded, he said, the national tuberculosis rate had fallen from 205 per 100,000 to just 60, but the need for places like Arequipa remained as crucial as before. By the time of Arequipa's twenty-fifth birthday, two more women-only sanatoria had been opened: Hill-crest, in Sunland, California, and the Sands House in Denver.

The day of the party, forty-three patients filled Arequipa's beds. Since 1920 the forty-bed capacity had stayed fairly static; by the mid-1930s, when the waiting list was always full, the staff managed to squeeze three more beds into the wards. This did not surprise Philip King Brown. He knew why women were still at risk for tuberculosis: poverty, unhealthful working conditions, and ignorance. And there was one more: women would always need sanatorium care, he believed, as long as they are "stupid enough to spend most of their lives dieting."[11]

He wasn't the only doctor who thought dieting put women on the road to getting TB. Dr. Owen felt the same, and in 1930 a San Francisco reporter sat her down for an interview that was carried in papers all over the country. Ethel Owen never minced words. "The woman of 40 can reduce with impunity," she said. "The woman of 20 undertakes a diet with the probability that she will be the prey of tuberculosis."[12] In 1930 women tried to lose weight for that flapper look. By 1936, when Philp King Brown ranted about dieting, the reason had more to do with Hollywood glamour and other impossible ideals.

A few months before Arequipa's anniversary party, Dr. Owen visited San Francisco radio stations to give ten-minute talks about TB prevention. The broadcasts were syndicated to stations in Portland, Oregon; Billings, Montana; Seattle, Washington; and Los Angeles. In addition to her duties as Arequipa's medical director she was supervisor of the child hygiene division of the San Francisco Department of Health and medical advisor to Stanford's school of nursing.

She was a busy woman and liked it that way. But sometime before the end of 1936, she resigned as Arequipa's medical director and Cabot Brown took over the duties that had once been his father's. Ethel Owen had worked at the sanatorium almost full-time for more than fifteen years, and she now wanted to concentrate on her work in public health for the city of San Francisco. Philip and Cabot Brown were grateful for what Ethel Owen had done for them and for Arequipa, and she and Adelaide stayed close for the rest of their lives.[13]

Her departure was also significant in another way: Ethel Owen was the last female doctor ever to work at Arequipa.

∽

Things were humming along at the sanatorium, so Philip King Brown was able to concentrate on a topic that was as important to him as TB prevention: health insurance for the poor.

His experience at the San Francisco Polyclinic, and with the women of Arequipa, showed him that death and disease followed the less fortunate, because they had no financial safety net. In making Arequipa affordable for working women, by enlisting charitable agencies to help women pay for their care, and by finding donors to allow the polyclinic to provide free services, Philip Brown was doing everything he could to get poor people the medical care they needed before they fell into pauperism.

He felt that American business had a part to play in this crusade. He had long been an attending physician at Southern Pacific Hospital in San Francisco, which was founded to treat railroad workers who had accidents or became ill. He felt that its programs of preventive medicine—which looked early for signs of disease in working men and treated them before they became debilitating—could be adapted on the state level for all types of workers.

As early as 1915 he had visited some of San Francisco's major employers, such as Levi Strauss & Co. and the Emporium department store, and given lunchtime talks on tuberculosis prevention to employees. He convinced some large corporations to subsidize the treatment of employees who had TB and needed to go to Arequipa. His rationale was this: paying for an employee to get sanatorium treatment so she could come back to work was more efficient and cost-effective in the long run than hiring someone new, who needed training and was an unknown quantity.

The Pacific States Telephone Company took Philip King Brown's ideas and made them into policy, sending a number of its operators to Arequipa over the course of two decades. In 1932, for example, a young woman operator who lived with her father became very ill. He did not believe in doctors, so she kept going to work and got progressively sicker. Her manager at Pacific Telephone recognized the symptoms of tuberculosis, thanks to Dr. Philip Brown's educational efforts. He contacted Arequipa and got the woman admitted; the company paid for her care. Not only did it take care of a valuable worker; she was also removed from the workplace so that she wouldn't infect everyone else.

In the years after World War I, the state of California tried to create insurance programs for the poor, both through general elections and putting bills through the legislature. Funding would come from employers and state subsidies, but from 1918 through the 1930s, nothing passed either the voters or the lawmakers. This didn't stop Philip King Brown from writing and speaking about the desperate need for health insurance and the need to lobby the California legislature to pass bills, which were refined and rewritten after each failure. At the same time, he also believed that private initiative had the power to get things done. That's exactly what he had accomplished with Arequipa, which more than twenty-five years later was fulfilling its original mission while keeping up with the latest advances in tuberculosis treatment.[14]

∾

Philip Brown's compassionate personality showed itself with friends as well as his patients. The family had a home at Lake Tahoe, on the California–Nevada border, and spent time with their lakeside neighbors. One of them was a young woman named Phoebe who was a student at Vassar in the 1930s. During one winter semester, she and some friends were skating on a frozen pond and one of the girls fell through a crack in the ice. Phoebe dove into the water to try to save her, but she had already drowned. Phoebe fell into a deep depression for the rest of the season and went to Tahoe the following summer to be with her family. Philip had heard about the accident and sought out the young woman for some long conversations. He helped her understand that the drowning was not her fault, and she went back to college without the heavy weight she had carried for so long.

Cabot Brown's son James wrote a memoir of his early life and said this about his grandfather: "It is easy for me to envision him, with his kindly countenance and already snow-white hair, in dialogue with Phoebe, asking her reassuring questions and offering sympathetic comments, always at just the right moment."[15]

Throughout 1939 and into 1940, Philip King Brown worked on his papers and speeches and enjoyed time with his expanding family. His three sons were married, and grandchildren had begun to arrive. Hillyer, the oldest, was a lawyer with the prestigious San Francisco firm Orrick, Palmer & Dahlquist. Bruce lived in Los Angeles and worked in the aircraft industry.

Daughter Phoebe Brown took another, more creative path. She studied English, architecture, and art at Bryn Mawr and got a BA in English from the University of California–Berkeley in 1932. She then took graduate courses in both English and architecture through 1935. In between her studies she embarked on a series of travels to Hawaii, Europe, New York, and the Caribbean, either with family members or by herself, including a year-long trip to Europe with her aunt Adelaide. In 1938 she went to the Turkish–Syrian border with archaeologist Arnold Walter Lawrence, brother of the famed T. E. Lawrence. She drew the plans of the crusader fortifications he excavated there. When she wasn't traveling, she lived with her parents in their home overlooking the Golden Gate.[16]

The family experienced losses too. Philip and Adelaide Brown's sister, Harriet Darling, had moved back to San Francisco from Boston after her husband died in 1920. She was living in Santa Clara, south of the city, when she passed away on May 31, 1935. She was the youngest child of Henry and Charlotte Brown, only sixty-four years old.

Like her mother, Dr. Adelaide Brown worked until she was no longer able. She was on the California Board of Public Health for decades and advocated for "well baby" clinics in San Francisco and around the Bay Area. She continued to work at her mother's hospital, traveled around Asia to observe health care for women and children there, and was a mentor for young female doctors who chose to become medical missionaries overseas. She continued to advocate for clean milk well into the 1930s and was one of the founders of Planned Parenthood in San Francisco. She closed her office in 1939, though many of her longtime patients still dropped in at her house when they needed care. She never turned them away.

She was also well-known for being something else: a reckless driver. All the parents who lived in her neighborhood instructed their children to get off the street when they saw Dr. Adelaide get into her car. (The dogs apparently scattered on their own.) After the Golden Gate and Bay Bridges were constructed, the city of San Francisco changed some street orientations to help with traffic flow; some became one-way only. One day, seventy-year-old Adelaide was driving the wrong way on one of these rerouted thoroughfares in downtown San Francisco and a motorcycle officer pulled her over. She berated him at the top of her voice, saying she had driven east on Pine Street all her life and wasn't going to change now. She then threatened to contact the chief of police, who was a friend of hers, but what happened after that did not make it into family lore. The woman who once chased a bear out of her tent with a broom did not get less fearless with age.

She and Philip were famous for holding vitriolic conversations at holiday dinners about San Francisco doctors they felt were less than fully competent. But Adelaide, like her brother, was also perceptive and capable of great compassion. She delivered Cabot Brown's second son, Stephen. (She was out of the country when the eldest son, James, was born.) When baby Philip was on his way in 1934, Cabot's wife, Peggy, went to Adelaide for a checkup. She noticed that the doctor seemed distracted and then noticed that she wrote down the wrong blood pressure numbers. Peggy was nervous about confronting Adelaide with her concerns, but she didn't have to. A short time later, Adelaide went to her and suggested that she find another physician for the duration of her pregnancy.

She realized she'd made an error during their appointment and didn't want the young woman to be uneasy. Nephew James later wrote that this was an act of "graciousness by a proud, very self-assured elder."[17]

In the summer of 1940, Phoebe Brown visited Mexico but took a plane home early, in the second week of July. Her beloved Aunt Adelaide had been ill for weeks, and it looked like she wasn't going to get better. She chose to remain at home rather than go to a hospital, and on July 29, 1940, Dr. Adelaide Brown died, at age seventy-two.

In late October that same year, Philip King Brown, suffering from stomach cancer, was quietly admitted to Stanford Hospital. Few people beyond the family were told. So it was a shock to his friends and colleagues when they learned of his death just a few days later, on October 28. His funeral was held the next day at the Brown family home.

The effect of his passing on Arequipa's staff, patients, and former patients can only be imagined. Patients remembered his calm presence, how he was outspoken about beating tuberculosis yet still sympathetic with their fears. Hundreds of women owed him their very lives, and some owed him their new professions. He had given female doctors and nurses a place to practice medicine and provided care to women who might otherwise have died or spent their lives suffering from chronic illnesses. No one recorded how these women felt about losing Philip King Brown. Had they been asked, they would likely have echoed what Dr. Langley Porter wrote in the obituary he published in the California Medical Association's journal.

Dr. Porter was dean of the school of medicine at the University of California in San Francisco, and he encompassed Philip King Brown's life and personality in just one description: "A man of high character, philanthropic disposition, a scholar of great attainment, a citizen whose self-sacrifice and services to the community were many and invaluable, a gentleman in every sense of the word."[18]

A few years after her husband's death, Helen Brown commissioned an artist to make a granite bench to honor Dr. Brown's work at Arequipa. His name was carved into the bench's back, and a bronze plaque with a poem by Bruce Porter was installed underneath it. On either side of the plaque were Brown's birth and death dates, and below this the words "Founder of Arequipa." The bench was placed just down the curved driveway from the sanatorium's front door, so that anyone coming or going could easily see it. The bronze plaque was stolen a few years after Helen died, and daughter Phoebe replaced it with a caduceus design rendered in colorful ceramic tile.

These were all fine and true tributes to Philip King Brown as physician and colleague. To his many former patients, however, he would always be "Daddy Brown."

Cabot Brown was now in charge of Arequipa, and he put his own stamp on the sanatorium, beginning with the staff. He had a thriving practice of his own in San Francisco and needed more visiting physicians to keep Arequipa running. He was lucky to find two volunteers right away.

Dr. Harry J. Pruett was the son of a prominent Fresno physician and earned his own MD at Stanford in 1917, when he was twenty-six years old. He began his practice in San Francisco and later married Alberta Morbia, who had a silver-plated family pedigree: she was the granddaughter of Adolph Sutro, who had made millions with his Sutro Tunnel, which moved excess water out of the mines in the famed Comstock Lode in Nevada, making extraction of the millions of dollars in silver much easier. He had also been mayor of San Francisco.

Dr. Pruett started working at Arequipa sometime in the mid-1930s.[19] In late 1940 Dr. Glenroy Pierce came on staff. Dr. Pierce was a generation younger than Pruett, born around 1912 in Georgia. He went to Stanford Medical School and earned his MD in 1937. By 1940 he was one of the physicians at the Arroyo Tuberculosis Sanatorium in Livermore, a rural town about forty-five miles east of San Francisco. He and his wife lived on the property, but around 1943 they left Arroyo and moved to San Francisco, where Pierce opened a private practice. A mutual interest in tuberculosis brought Dr. Pierce and Cabot Brown together, and he was soon making a weekly trip to Arequipa.[20]

So was Dr. Lloyd Dickey. Dr. Ethel Owen had brought him onto the staff when she was the medical director and the main attending physician. Dickey had earned his medical degree in the Midwest but came to California in 1923 to intern at Stanford University. A few years later he was one of Stanford's professors, head of the Pediatrics Department, and chief of the university's children's clinic in San Francisco. In the early 1930s he met Cabot Brown, who asked him if he would work as a visiting physician at Arequipa with a very specific group of patients. They were his specialty and were the most vulnerable of all: children.[21]

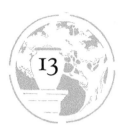

MAGIC BULLETS

PHILIP KING BROWN STARTED ADMITTING CHILDREN to the sanatorium around 1932 because there were very few "preventoriums" in the Bay Area for them to go to. These were country properties, much like Elizabeth Ashe's Hill Farm, but their sole purpose was to keep children from getting tuberculosis. Dr. Brown did send some young people to Hill Farm in the first few years after Arequipa opened—children who were either at risk of getting TB or who needed a place to stay for a few months because their mothers were taking the cure at the sanatorium. Brown was deeply grateful to Elizabeth Ashe for her help as he struggled to get Arequipa going.

But Hill Farm wasn't a true preventorium, which was a kind of medical summer camp, overseen by a trained TB nurse or physician. Kids lived the outdoor life while being monitored by doctors and nurses, and fed to bursting just like adults taking the rest cure. But no state had enough preventoriums to help with the volume of cases that showed up in doctors' waiting rooms, and conditions during the Depression made things worse.

Only two preventoriums were within driving distance of San Francisco: one in Livermore and the other in San Mateo, just south of the city.[1] They did not have enough beds to meet what Dr. Brown saw as a critical need, so he decided to make room for girls at Arequipa.

Having children in the wards was an emotional boost for the women, who didn't get to see their own very often. Entertainments aimed specifically at little girls became part of the regular programs of outside amusements. In November 1932, for example, a few members of the Young Ladies' Institute, a Catholic charity from San Francisco, went to Arequipa and performed a play called *School Days*, which also involved singing, dancing, and recitation.

Child patients trickled in and were discharged throughout the rest of the decade. In 1940 a fourteen-year-old girl from the farming town of Watsonville was carried through the doors and placed gently into a bed in the downstairs ward. Her name was Rose.

Rose's ancestors were Cantonese and had come to the United States from China before the restrictions of the 1882 Chinese Exclusion Act. Born in June 1926 in San Francisco, she was the youngest of six, with four sisters and one brother (the eldest) ahead of her. Her grandfather owned an apple drying facility in Watsonville, and her father was an itinerant worker, sometimes following the fruit around California or working in restaurants. At some point in Rose's early childhood, the family moved to Watsonville. She and her siblings attended the local public school and also spent a few afternoons and a Saturday each week at the Chinese school, learning their family's first language.

When Rose was thirteen, her mother died of tuberculosis. Six months later the school nurse noticed that Rose was out sick for days at a time, and even when she came to class she had worrisome symptoms. Officials were always on the lookout for TB in their students, which is what the nurse suspected. A local doctor confirmed it: Rose had TB in both lungs and had to leave school immediately. Bed rest at home would be helpful, but what she really needed was time in a sanatorium. The doctor knew about Arequipa and that it took in children, so he made the arrangements for Rose to be admitted. A few days after she celebrated her fourteenth birthday, Rose's brother and the school nurse drove her to Arequipa.

She was so sick that she didn't get out of bed for four years. "My feet didn't touch the floor that whole time," she remembered. She had to be carried to the bathroom and the treatment rooms, a task that fell to two young Filipino American stewards, who crossed their arms to make a type of chair for any patient who wasn't ambulatory.

Like all the other TB patients, she had to wolf down piles of food three times a day. She ate so many potatoes that her brother started calling her Spuds. She also drank a lot of milk, which was not a big part of her diet at home. But even with all these calories, she lost weight when she first entered Arequipa. The doctors decided to give her pneumothorax right away. They also gave her extra food, mostly rice with lots of butter, and she soon gained a few pounds.

Rose's new world was strange, but she was so ill that she just surrendered to the doctors, the nurses, and whatever they needed to do to her. "In those days you did what you were told, you didn't think for yourself," as she put it. Philip King Brown would have approved of this attitude.

Dr. Dickey was in charge of the children's treatment, even though Cabot Brown and the other physicians also looked in on the young patients during their visiting days. Rose remembered him as a bashful fuddy-duddy and a natural pediatrician. He usually went to Arequipa on Fridays, taking the ferry from San Francisco and the train to the whistle-stop down the road from the sanatorium. Emma Applegren would pick him up. He would do his rounds with both the child and the adult patients and then have lunch before taking the train and the ferry back across the bay.

Dickey and most other commuters were glad when the Golden Gate Bridge opened in 1937, because they could now drive directly to destinations north of the city. But they mourned the loss of the enjoyable ferry rides, which gave travelers a unique way to get around. The night of the last ferry journey, Dr. Dickey, an attorney friend, and an insurance executive, who generally traveled on the same boat, got off on the Marin County side and went straight to the nearest bar to toast the end of an era.[2]

~

A new visiting physician named Thomas Wiper took a special interest in Rose's care. Wiper was born in South Dakota in 1904 and got his MD from Stanford in 1931, serving a residency at San Francisco General Hospital. They were "rivals for my affection," she remembered, which was another way of saying that they knew how sick she was. They conspired between them to keep Rose alive and also gave her nicknames: Roses (Dr. Brown) and Rosie (Dr. Wiper). Dr. Wiper had a beautiful garden at his Marin County home, and when he visited on Mondays, he always brought gigantic bouquets of begonias for Arequipa's flower vases, making sure that Rose had some for herself.

Once she started gaining weight and feeling better, Rose paid more attention to her surroundings and to the women in the other beds. The girls were not separated from the adults in the ward, so Rose got to know patients of all ages. One was a Japanese American woman named Mary who was studying to be a teacher at San Francisco State College when she got sick. She was already an up patient when Rose was admitted and spent a lot of time wandering the ward talking to the other patients. She had a soft voice and a quiet laugh but was also a lot of fun. She addressed Rose as Toots.

Dolores, nicknamed Donnie, was in the bed next to Rose. Her condition was bad enough that she had needed thoracoplasty—the removal of a few ribs to permanently collapse the lung—so one of her shoulders was permanently higher than the other. Gertrude, a willowy blond, was a health nut and would put wheat germ in Rose's orange juice. Rose didn't like it, but the staff didn't seem to mind what Gertrude was doing.

There was also a minor celebrity among the ranks. A girl named Mary, about Rose's age, was the niece of famed Chinese American nightclub owner Charlie Low. His Forbidden City club opened in 1938 just outside the gate that separated Chinatown from downtown San Francisco. It featured a collection of Asian women who performed tame but still titillating musical numbers for mainly white audiences, which sometimes included movie stars such as Ronald Reagan. The fathers, brothers, and other male relatives of some of Arequipa's patients probably dropped in at Forbidden City now and then too. Mary gave Rose a photo of herself, which she signed, "To my best friend Rose."

Rose's ward mates showered her with birthday cards when she turned sixteen. The card from Gertrude read, "Many Many happy returns of this day to Dr. Wiper's 'sweetheart' and our beloved Rose."

Keeping the patients cheered and optimistic was still an important part of the cure. On December 18, 1941, as the country was still reeling from the attack on Pearl Harbor, the local Camp Fire Girls made corsages for all Arequipa's patients to wear at the sanatorium's Christmas celebrations. Less than a quarter century after "the war to end all wars," a global conflict reached in to change Arequipa again.

In 1942 Dr. Cabot Brown enlisted in the U.S. Naval Reserve Medical Corps. He spent a short time at the Oakland Naval Hospital and then served on naval hospital ships in the Pacific, where he got the occasional leave to see Bob Hope on landlocked U.S. installations. Dr. Wiper worked for the army at Halloran General Hospital in Staten Island and then as chief of the thoracic surgical service for the army in Spokane.

Dr. Pruett, age fifty when the war began, stayed on as a visiting physician at Arequipa. Dr. Pierce was thirty but was 4-F (unfit for military service) because of a leg problem that gave him a permanent limp, so he also continued his work for Dr. Brown. With their help, Emma Applegren kept Arequipa afloat during the war years. Like his father, Cabot knew that the sanatorium was in good hands during his absence, even when those hands belonged to a woman. And both doctors sent letters to patients while they were gone.

In 1943 two Latina sisters from Napa, Josephine and Gabriella, were admitted to Arequipa; Josephine was eleven and Gabriella a few years younger. By the spring of 1945 Josephine was well enough to go home and was waiting for her official discharge. Before she left she wandered the wards, soliciting money from the adults, and collected $100, which she gave to the Marin County headquarters of the Red Cross War Fund. Gabriella was sent home a few months later, and she spent the time after her sister's departure making surgical dressings, which were sent to the front.

The war years brought both sorrow and intrigue to the Brown family. Helen Hillyer Brown, Philip's beloved wife and the mother of Hillyer, Cabot, Phoebe, and Bruce, died at her home on May 31, 1944, while Cabot was still at sea. Phoebe Brown was also away; during the war she worked for the Office of Strategic Services in China, Burma, and India. Although she always said she was just a file clerk, hints of special work (spying) for America's first intelligence-gathering agency followed her for decades. And she dropped hints to her family that she became friends with another woman employed by the OSS: Julia Child. No one named for Phoebe Hearst could have an ordinary life.[3]

Very little news about the war filtered into Arequipa, or the adults just didn't talk about it in front of the girls. Rose therefore didn't find it strange that a Japanese American woman was being treated there, as Mary was still at Arequipa when the war began. If Mary's family had been sent to an internment camp, she didn't mention it. Rose says she never heard anyone say anything anti-Japanese, either—at least not to Mary's face.

Rose never thought herself the target of racist comments, though some of the remarks she heard are jarring to today's ears. One nurse would occasionally refer to a "Chinaman" when she was taking Rose's temperature or changing her sheets and then laugh as she walked away. One year a fellow patient sent her a birthday card that ended, "Good luck, long life and prosperity to my little fugitive from a Chinese laundry." This casual racism, normal for the 1940s, went over Rose's head, and she said she never felt ostracized or threatened.

After four years on strict bed rest, Rose was granted an up and moved to the ambulatory ward, where she continued to get stronger. She was nearly eighteen years old and Emma Applegren was worried about her future, since she had not been able to attend high school. The other girls in her ward only spent a few months or at most a year at Arequipa, so they could make up their class time more easily. When Rose was on bed rest, she was too sick to muster the strength to read, but once Rose was an up patient, Emma decided that something had to be done about her education. She found a teacher in nearby San Rafael who was willing to come out to Arequipa and give Rose some basic lessons. She gave Rose reading and grammar workbooks, and though they only spent a semester together, it was obvious to the teacher that Rose was bright and motivated. She would soon be proved right.

By early 1945 Rose was no longer contagious and didn't need any more pneumothorax treatments. Other patients with this diagnosis would have been getting ready to return home. But Rose didn't have a home to go to. Her father was still an itinerant worker, and her siblings had married and were scattered around the state. She was now nineteen but did not have the resources to support herself.

The staff knew Rose very well by now and could tell she was a smart young woman. So, after exchanging letters with the still-overseas Cabot Brown, Emma Applegren started to give Rose some work to do around the sanatorium, to keep her occupied and to pay her a little money. This also allowed the medical staff to keep an eye on her and to make sure her symptoms didn't return. Rose traded her bathrobe for dresses and skirts, as well as new stockings and shoes. Her family didn't have the money to pay for new outfits, so Applegren dug into her own purse to buy clothes and accessories for Arequipa's newest and youngest employee.

Donnie had taught her Gregg shorthand, and Rose taught herself to type during her up days, so she already had some useful skills. She did a bit of typing and bookkeeping in the office, and then the nurses taught her how to collect sputum samples, take blood, and work in the lab, dyeing the samples to check for TB bacilli. They also taught her to clean and sharpen the needles for the pneumothorax machine and put them into the autoclave to be sterilized.

Another former patient, Frieda Craig, was now the lab tech, and she and Rose became friends as well as coworkers. In addition to doing clerical work, Rose worked half days in the lab, emptied bedpans, and swept the wards. The doctors and nurses had, in effect, created a combination of occupational therapy, job training, and charity just for her. Cabot Brown no doubt approved; he once wrote her a letter from his posting in the Pacific that said, "I hear you're running the place."

Since Rose wasn't a patient anymore, the staff rigged up a bed for her in a little room off the downstairs ward. Mice skittered in the walls of the thirty-year-old building, and she would bang on the panel next to her bed at night to keep them quiet. She ate the same food as the patients and kept her weight up, and she enjoyed talking with her friends who were still getting treatment. She was very happy when Cabot Brown returned to the Bay Area just days after the Japanese surrender in August 1945, though she didn't see as much of him now that she was no longer a patient.

Emma Applegren had been especially sweet to Rose when she was a patient, and she and Rose, despite their age difference, became true friends the longer Rose stayed at Arequipa. Applegren lived in a cottage behind the sanatorium; a path connected the two buildings. Her two dogs, Ladye Buffe Craig and Ladye Heather Lumsden, would always start yipping whenever Applegren walked to her cottage, which everyone in the sanatorium could hear. Although the dogs were sometimes allowed into the wards under Philip King Brown's administration, Cabot made Arequipa dog-free when he was in charge.

On Rose's twenty-first birthday, in June 1947, Applegren ordered the cook (who happened to be her sister, Pauline) to make fried chicken for everyone to honor Rose's big day. A few months later, seven years after she entered Arequipa as a desperately ill child, Rose was discharged as cured. However, she didn't go far.

Dr. Thomas Wiper gave up his visiting physician duties at Arequipa after the war. He and two other San Francisco physicians purchased the California Sanatorium in Belmont, which had opened just a year before Arequipa did. Wiper was the medical director and had kept in touch with Rose during and after his war service. When he heard she was getting ready to leave Arequipa, he offered her a permanent job and a room in the nurse's dormitory if she wanted it. She had learned so many skills during her time at Arequipa that she could probably have found a job in a laboratory or an office anywhere, but she chose to stay with Dr. Wiper. She would test the waters of the wider world in a familiar place.[4]

In the months after Dr. Philip King Brown's death, Arequipa's patients, staff, doctors, and nurses continued to tread the routine he had set up nearly thirty years before. To follow the rules to the letter was to feel him walking the wards again, if only in spirit. Cabot Brown did the same, and with full authority over staffing and patients, he could have started admitting men to Arequipa if he chose to. But he believed in his father's vision of a women-only sanatorium and kept true to Arequipa's mission. He also knew that mixing the sexes in a sanatorium would make his job a lot harder.

Most sanatoria in the United States treated both men and women and constructed separate wards or even separate buildings for male and female patients, not to mention separate bathrooms and dining rooms. The 1914 *Tuberculosis Hospital and Sanatorium Construction* manual has drawings of various sanatorium designs, with everything from walkways to full-size structures separating the men's and women's cottages or wards. Tuberculosis treatment was the same for both men and women, so that was not the reason to keep the genders apart. Modesty and privacy were big issues. But doctors also knew that mixing the sexes was a potential powder keg of repressed desires, competition, and emotional upsets, none of which were helpful in the TB cure.

In 1948 writer Betty MacDonald published *The Plague and I*, a memoir of her TB treatment at Firland Sanatorium in Seattle (though she called the sanatorium The Pines in the book). She included a story about the anticipation of being wheeled into an auditorium one evening to see a film alongside the elusive male patients from other buildings. A nurse threw cold water on her enthusiasm, however. "You will be called for by a *male* (she said male in a low throbbing voice as though it were some dangerous new sex) ambulant patient but you are not to speak to or to laugh with your escort."

MacDonald wrote that she was chagrined when a terrified teenager called for her, and she was not surprised when she saw that the men were placed on one side of the auditorium with the women far away on the other. The open space between the groups was "carefully patrolled by gimlet-eyed nurses with powerful flashlights to make sure that the sexes didn't mingle in the dark." The sanatorium's administration nevertheless decided that the evening's entertainment would be the 1936 romantic drama *Camille*, in which a pale Greta Garbo plays a woman who eventually dies of tuberculosis.[5]

Both Cabot Brown and his father knew about the hazards of mingling the sexes in a sanatorium setting. While separate wards had been built on Arequipa's two different floors and double wings, it would have been hard to keep men and women apart, especially when all the beds were full. The wards were designed so that doctors and nurses could move easily between them, and this would have given male and female up patients plenty of opportunity for romance or its opposite.

More male faces were on hand after 1940, though. Cabot Brown, Lloyd Dickey, Harry Pruett, and Glenroy Pierce were now the full medical staff, and for the rest of Arequipa's institutional life, no more women doctors would work Arequipa's wards.

Why was this? Was this deliberate on Cabot's part? Did he prefer to work with male doctors? Or perhaps the "female doctor" was less of an anomaly now, and women didn't feel the need to prove themselves by overcommitting and adding the job of visiting physician to their regular practices, as Emma Willits, Mary Mentzer, and Ethel Owen had done. Other women had filled in when the main female medicos were unavailable, but their service was transitory. Perhaps Cabot just didn't have the professional contacts with female physicians that his father had.

Whatever the reason, all of Cabot's decisions were based on one premise: Arequipa was his baby. He loved spending time with the patients and was so proud of the sanatorium that he even invited some doctors from Arequipa, Peru, for a visit.[6]

It seems counterintuitive, but Arequipa was still a destination—and not just for those who came to visit patients. Doctors held meetings there, entertainers shared their talents, and friends of the staff dropped by for lunch or dinner as if the sanatorium were a private home. Arequipa's appeal makes sense. The building itself was beautiful, and its little valley was an oasis of quiet in an increasingly strident world. Marin County was becoming an important suburb of San Francisco, with more people moving into its towns, freeways being expanded, and new subdivisions on the drawing board. Arequipa really was a place of rest, even for those who didn't have TB.

Postwar progress extended into medicine too. Bacteriologists made discoveries that gave life back to gravely wounded soldiers, the ironic positive side of war. These scientists would also profoundly alter the lives of the stenographers, housewives, telephone operators, students, and teachers at Arequipa, and the men and women in the beds of every sanatorium and hospital tuberculosis ward in America.

From Arequipa's opening in 1911 to the death of Dr. Philip King Brown in 1940, the pace of innovation in America hit fast forward. In the space of a generation, inventions modernized travel, communication, construction, and food, and dazzled consumers. Among these inventions were the electric traffic light, the radio altimeter, liquid propellant, Formica, hydraulic brakes, nylon, and Teflon. The American diet was enriched, though not especially improved, by the introduction of the fortune cookie, the Eskimo Pie, and the corn dog. The pop-up toaster made breakfast easier to make, and the electric guitar would soon revolutionize music.

Medicine also had some big breakthroughs, from the Band-Aid to the iron lung. The biggest news in the doctor's office was the discovery of what German biochemist Paul Ehrlich called "magic bullets": chemical serums to treat specific diseases that had destroyed lives for centuries. Salvarsan (introduced in 1909) was the first real cure for syphilis and was also considered the first chemotherapy drug.

In 1928 Scottish bacteriologist Alexander Fleming was working with deadly staphylococci and discovered that a mold growing on some cultures actually killed the bacteria. He then experimented with what he called "mold juice" and in 1929 introduced penicillin, which was dubbed an antibiotic. It not only killed the staph infection but was also effective against scarlet fever, pneumonia, diphtheria, and meningitis.

From the 1930s to the early 1940s, French microbiologist René Dubos, working at the Rockefeller Institute for Medical Research, took this concept into new realms. He synthesized a new drug called tyrothricin, which became the first commercially available antibiotic. His work helped create more interest in uses for penicillin and antibiotics in general.

But even in the midst of all of this newness in daily life and medicine, one thing remained the same: there was no treatment for tuberculosis. No magic bullet or mold killed the tubercle bacillus, and Arequipa, along with every other sanatorium in America, continued to admit patients for the rest cure, even though TB rates had been declining.

In 1900 tuberculosis was the second leading cause of death in the United States, with 194 deaths per 100,000 individuals; by 1940 the death rate had plunged to just 46 per 100,000. The reason for these good numbers is very simple. The early to mid–twentieth century brought improvements in food safety and cleanliness, public sanitation, and housing; tuberculosis had few places to hide when a child's milk was free of bovine bacillus, spitting was outlawed, and new housing was built in major cities.

TB still lurked, of course. With the success of salvarsan and penicillin in mind, biochemists looked for ways to synthesize new antibiotics to treat other diseases, including tuberculosis. One of the scientists was Ukrainian-born Selman Waksman, who was working at Rutgers University in the early 1940s. His graduate students Albert Schatz, Elizabeth Bugie, and H. Christine Reilly labored to isolate a soil-based bacterium named *Streptomyces griseus*, which they believed could be even more powerful than penicillin.

In 1943 Waksman and his students refined the bacterium into a drug called streptomycin. In 1944 it was used in a clinical trial with a desperately ill TB patient, whose swift improvement astonished even the drug's creators. By 1945 streptomycin was widely available to doctors and being handed out to tubercular men and women all over the United States.

The discovery was a mixed bag though. Research showed that the drug was most effective when it was used with long-standing traditional treatments: rest, good food, and fresh air. Doctors also noticed that the TB bacillus started to develop a resistance to streptomycin after just a few months, though this amount of time was often enough to get TB patients back on their feet, as long as they followed good health guidelines at home.

A remedy for streptomycin's drawbacks soon came out of Denmark. In the early years of World War II a biochemist named Jörgen Lehmann had developed a solution called para-aminosalicylic acid, which was very effective against a range of bacterial infections, including tuberculosis. However, like streptomycin, it was not a complete cure and the body quickly developed a resistance.

After the war, Waksman, Lehman, and other researchers began to correspond about their work, and after many rounds of clinical trials, they realized that the two drugs in combination were more powerful than each drug on its own. By 1948 they had developed a combination therapy called isoniazid, and to the great joy of doctors everywhere, it turned out to be the magic bullet they were looking for. For the first time since Robert Koch discovered the tubercle bacillus and Dr. Edward Trudeau opened the first American sanatorium, doctors could use the words *cure* and *tuberculosis* together and really mean it.[7]

In April 1947 Cabot Brown gave streptomycin to an Arequipa patient for the first time, watching her progress over the course of four months. This was not an unexpected development. Another patient wrote about the impact of the drug's discovery on everyone at the sanatorium: "We first started reading news releases on the expectations of the new 'wonder' drug to cure T.B., made from an earthen mold called streptomycin in early 1946. Every patient read every available word and our hopes were high. In the fall of '46 tubercular war veterans were given priority & optional use of all available strepto. As more of the drug was released we anxiously awaited its use at Arequipa."

She then reported on what happened to patients who took the first strepto: "Yes, the girl gained weight, bug diminished and calcification increased."

The antibiotic was the biggest news of 1947 at Arequipa, along with construction of a new building for the nurses. They had been living in cottages on the property, but Cabot Brown decided they needed their own, nicer dormitory. He hired architect Gardner A. Dailey to design the structure, even though John Bakewell, the original architect, was still alive and practicing. But Cabot put his own stamp on what was now his sanatorium, and he preferred the designs of the more modernist Dailey. The patients, however, had a different opinion. According to one, "Mother Applegren let us look at the plans—of course we didn't like them."[8]

Cabot Brown believed that drugs had a place in TB treatment, but when women came to Arequipa it was to take the rest cure. If he thought a patient would be helped by taking streptomycin, he prescribed it for her, but he never gave up on the power of the sanatorium. Even as the end of the 1940s approached, and the news of what isoniazid was doing for TB patients was making the news, he kept Arequipa's beds filled.

From the earliest days of sanatorium treatment in the United States, doctors had a special worry about their female patients: pregnancy. Carrying a child to term while taking the TB cure was dangerous for both mother and baby. As far back as the 1920s, doctors argued about whether pregnant women should even be admitted to sanatoria and, if they were, how their treatment was supposed to differ from that of the other patients. Months of rest were not incompatible with a successful pregnancy, but if any complications arose, the patient would have to go to another hospital, and this would put her own cure behind schedule. Sanatoria did not have delivery rooms, so pregnant patients also went to nearby hospitals when they went into labor.

These policies were not consistent across all sanatoria. Some institutions asked women to leave once they were five or six months along, and some took pregnant women only if they could not be cared for at home. Others welcomed women in the early stages of both TB and pregnancy so that the health of both mother and baby could be watched and managed.

Tuberculosis shadowed the happy expectation of a baby's arrival. The strain of childbirth could tear open any healed-over cavities in the mother's lungs, and the bacillus could also be transmitted to the child through the umbilical cord or amniotic fluid. Breast feeding was actually safe, but the risk of the mother spreading droplets of the bacillus through her breath, holding a baby close, meant that little ones were often taken from their mothers immediately after birth.

Most doctors told pregnant tubercular patients who were less than three months along to get an abortion. Women who had recently left a sanatorium and became pregnant got the same advice, because hormonal and immune system changes could cause a flare-up of the disease and even mask its symptoms, so a pregnant woman might not even know she was infected. Abortion was illegal, of course, except in the rare cases when carrying a child to term could put the mother at risk. Having TB or being newly recovered from TB were unquestioned risks. Abortion was a fraught subject, something that was rarely openly discussed, and women agonized about the decision, even when doctors said it was necessary, legal, and safe.[9]

Cabot Brown and the other doctors at Arequipa regularly and rather firmly told tubercular pregnant women that they needed to abort before they could get treatment. In 1949 one of them was a Marin County woman named Patty (a pseudonym).

∾

In the 1940s the National Tuberculosis Association began to fund mobile X-ray trucks, which showed up at schools, stores, and businesses. There, people could get a free TB examination if they were worried about sudden symptoms of fatigue, coughing, or night sweats. Much of the funding came from the sale of Christmas Seals, a tradition dating back to 1907.

The idea of selling seals or stamps to help struggling sanatoria or individual TB patients began in Denmark in 1904. Three years later a woman named Emily Bissell, who worked for the Red Cross, heard about this idea and decided to adapt it to help raise money for a TB hospital in Delaware, selling the colorful stamps during the Christmas season.

The sale was a big success, especially after President Theodore Roosevelt endorsed the idea. The first batch sold out in two days. The Red Cross then took over the program and created a national, annual campaign called Christmas Seals. Artists vied with one another to design the stamps, and the sales funded anti-TB efforts in both states and counties. The Red Cross ran the program for twelve years, and in 1919 the National Tuberculosis Association took over, expanding its reach even further, including providing funds for cities to buy mobile X-ray units for TB screening.[10]

In October 1949 Patty got an X-ray at one of Marin County's mobile units. A few days after Thanksgiving, her doctor came to the house to tell her she had tuberculosis and to go right to bed. A couple of weeks later she got more news: she was pregnant. Dr. Glenroy Pierce, now the head physician at Arequipa, also made a house call. He said that a bed could be held for her at the sanatorium but that her condition was so advanced that she needed to terminate her pregnancy before she could be admitted. She was appalled when he told her she had a cavity the size of a walnut in one of her lungs.

Patty had many misgivings about aborting her baby, but she already had two children, whose health had to be her main concern. So she went to San Rafael General Hospital on December 27, 1949, for an abortion, and the next day her husband drove her to Arequipa.

By the time Patty was taking her cure, Dr. Cabot Brown had changed how the women progressed through their treatment. From 1911 until after World War II, a patient was admitted and given a bed, and she stayed put until she was considered cured (or, less frequently, until she died). But after the war, Cabot Brown decided to cluster women together based on their conditions. The sickest patients, the ones new to Arequipa, lived on the second-floor ward. Once their temperatures stayed steady, their cavities healed over, and they were granted their ups, they moved to the lower ward, where they could walk to the bathrooms and the dining room. When they were close to discharge, they were moved to a ground-floor ward called the Wing.

Patty went straight upstairs when she entered Arequipa. Fifteen women comprised the "sick ward" when she first arrived, and her fellow patients were an interesting mix of backgrounds and personalities. Patty kept a journal during her time at Arequipa. She was an outspoken woman who didn't pull punches about her fellow patients, the staff, or the sanatorium routine, which she likened to prison, however voluntary it was. And she had a lot to say about her wardmates.

Two of the women were Nisei, first-generation Japanese Americans, and it's revealing of Patty's own personality that she had no harsh words for them just four years after the end of World War II. Then there was Elli, a twenty-two-year-old war bride from Germany. Patty wrote about Elli's hard life in Berlin and how she had lost her father to tuberculosis just a few months earlier. She held little rancor for this representative of the Axis powers. But she didn't like Ellie personally, calling her a "selfish pig."

Lottie was a rugged gal who had bummed all over the country, and Paloma was originally from Tahiti. The other women came from all over California, as well as Oregon and Arizona. Some were married, others single, some teetering on being deserted by their husbands. Some later died.

Patty liked Dr. Cabot Brown and thought Emma Applegren was a lovely woman. But she didn't have many good things to say about Dr. Glenroy Pierce. He and his wife lived in Marin County, where the doctor had a garden he was very proud of. Some days when he came to do his rounds at Arequipa, he wore a jacket over his gardening clothes. He was abrupt with the patients, and Patty thought he was irritated at being pulled away from his yard.

One of the Japanese American women was named Kay, and she died in February 1950. Tuberculosis had taken over her intestines as well as her lungs, and she was so sick that Dr. Brown didn't want to move her to a hospital. The staff made her a bed in one of the back offices, and her husband came to see her every night to hold her hand. She lasted a week after she was moved, and then was gone.

Patty was very affected by Kay's death. But, like the other patients before her, she needed to concentrate on her own health, so she filled most of her journal with information on her X-rays, sputum tests, and how wonderful it was to use a real bathroom once she had been given an up.

A few other things were new under Cabot Brown's administration. Unlike in earlier decades, the women didn't have to put newspapers between the floor and the box springs of their beds when it was cold. Available to them was another recent invention: the electric blanket. But the wards were still open to the elements, and in winter ice sometimes covered the water pitchers in the morning.

Food, however, was the same as always: calorie-laden and heavy on dairy. The women occasionally got an unusual treat. The hills around Arequipa teemed with black-tailed deer, many of which encountered the rising tide of automobile traffic along Marin County's roads and ended up as road kill. Emma Applegren knew a few local hunters and arranged for them to field-dress some of the deer and send the meat to the sanatorium. Then everyone had venison for dinner. The hunters also sometimes brought extra deer meat of their own up to the sanatorium.

Patty stayed in the upper ward until the beginning of April 1950, when she was moved to the lower ward. Dr. Cabot Brown and Emma Applegren told her how well she was doing, and even earlier, in March, when she was getting an X-ray, Cabot Brown had said he could tell she was better just by looking at her. She was very happy about these developments but was self-aware enough to occasionally examine her own emotional state. She seemed to understand how little irritations could become massive annoyances in the confines of a bed in a TB ward. But deeper emotions lurked.

Unlike Lois Downey, whose toddler son could visit and even sit on her bed when she took the cure in the late 1920s, Patty could not welcome her children inside. She was allowed to talk to them only through a window when they came to visit. Standing on the pavement next to the sanatorium building, slightly embarrassed by the whole thing, her boy and girl didn't know what to do, but everyone soon broke the ice, and Patty thrilled to their voices.

On Easter Sunday in 1950 she called the children at home to hear what the Easter Bunny had brought them. At first she couldn't tell what her son was saying, and she panicked, thinking that she had been away from him so long that she couldn't understand him anymore. But she then realized that he had a mouthful of candy. Her daughter tried to pin her down about when she was coming home, and Patty managed to mollify her by saying that she had to wait until the weather was nice and warm.

Like her fellow patients, Patty was cheered a little by the presence of the children in the wards. Three or four of them were in beds at Arequipa when Patty was there. A local Girl Scout troop dropped by regularly to visit a couple of girls who had been Scouts before they got TB. When the Scouts came in to sing carols during Christmas in 1949, they met a new patient named Rose, who was just ten years old. They spent time with her again on Valentine's Day the following year, when they brought handmade decorations for everyone's meal tray. They then decided to do something to make Rose's life more interesting, so in March they dropped by and presented her with a Girl Scout handbook. With the help of the other girls, Rose began to do projects that wouldn't interfere with her cure. She was soon a member in good standing of Troop 71.

There was another death in the third week of April 1950. A woman named Mae, who was in the Wing and getting close to discharge, was preparing to get a procedure called a bronchoscopy, in which the doctors used a scope to take a look at the bronchial tubes. Patients gargled with an anesthetic such as Novocain or procaine first, and a "bronc" was considered a pretty routine examination. But on this day something went wrong.

As soon as she began to gargle, Mae blacked out and began convulsing. Her throat constricted and she died before doctors could do anything to help her. The whole sanatorium went into shock. Mae had been allergic to the anesthetic, but no one knew it. Even though it was just a terrible accident, Patty told the doctors that if they wanted to do a bronc on her, they would have to test her for allergies first.

Losing Mae was bad enough. But two days later, when Patty got the good news that she was being moved to the Wing, she was put into Mae's bed. She was worried that this would happen, but she knew that if the bed was filled, it would be good for everyone's morale. Her troubled mind did find compensations though. The Wing had large windows with a view of the road, and Patty could watch the cars go by and see who was coming up the drive.

Her sunny attitude soon began to wane. By early May she was restless, fed up with TB, fed up with trying to keep her morale high. At the end of the month she told Cabot Brown she was leaving because her family needed her. He wasn't happy about it, but he understood. He had been treating TB patients long enough to know that at a certain point, unhappiness with institutional living could stop the healing process in its tracks. He gave Patty a short lecture about how to take care of herself and then sent her joyfully home.[11]

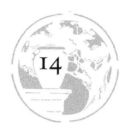

DANCING BACK TO BED

AS THE 1950S OPENED, Arequipa was functioning well but looked shabby. Again. The last time the buildings had been spruced up or renovated was 1932, and nearly twenty years on they needed structural work beyond new paint or flooring. Luckily, a woman on Cabot Brown's board of directors was as influential and socially minded as the women who had helped his father build Arequipa nearly forty years earlier.

Her name was Alice Kent. She was born Alice Cooke in Hawaii, the great-granddaughter of missionaries. Her father was a banker and politician, and the family was one half of Castle & Cooke, a conglomerate that had interests in Hawaiian sugar and pineapple plantations. The company also had part ownership of Matson Navigation, which pioneered luxury liner travel between California and Hawaii in the early years of the twentieth century. Alice was educated in Italy and at Vassar, and in 1929 she met a young man from Marin County who was visiting a friend in the islands.

He was Roger Kent, whose father, William, had served on Arequipa's board of trustees in the early years. Roger's mother, Elizabeth, was a prominent and tireless worker for women's suffrage. Roger grew up on the family estate in Marin County in the area now called Kent Woodlands (the nearby town of Kentfield is also named for the family), took a law degree, and became a leader in Democratic Party politics in California. He was as service-minded as his father, and in Alice he found an equally philanthropic partner. They were married in 1930 and had four children, though they lost one son to an accident when he was a child.

As she raised her family, Alice turned the Kent estate into a center for Marin County politics and philanthropy. The Kents hosted speakers from and held fund-raisers for the American Friends Service Committee, the American Civil Liberties Union, the Marin County Humane Society, and many other organizations. By 1949 Alice's interests had turned to the work of the National Tuberculosis Association, and she was named chairman of the Red Cross Christmas Seal drive that year. She held a tea at her home to thank all her volunteers once the drive was over.[1]

She was also on Arequipa's board of directors by this time. She knew everything about the sanatorium, including its problems. So in June 1951 she called together thirty-five society friends who had served with her on various committees or held events in their own homes. Five of them were also on Arequipa's board. Kent gave them lunch and told them that Arequipa needed their help, and by the time dessert was served, the women had come up with plans for a fund-raising dinner dance. In August the local newspaper, the *Daily Independent-Journal*, reported that the event was planned for September 15 and had both a theme and a name: A Night in Peru.

Alice Kent and her friends knew how to plan a party, and fifteen hundred people showed up at her home on a stunning September evening to enjoy themselves and contribute to a local cause. The house had a swimming pool and an outdoor dance pavilion, both of which were pressed into service. Masses of flowers and a South Pacific–style raft floated on the water. The dancing went on into the early morning under a lighted canopy. A few nights before the dinner, the Kents hosted a cocktail party for some San Francisco doctors and other special guests, so they could learn about Arequipa before the main event. And Kent went even further to help Arequipa: any staff member not on duty the night of the dinner was welcome to come as her guest.

A Night in Peru was a smash. Alice Kent not only secured her standing as Marin County's premier hostess, but she also had the satisfaction of knowing that her efforts raised $10,000 for Arequipa, worth about $100,000 today. She was pleased at the results but knew that the sanatorium needed more than that to make the necessary renovations and repairs.

Meanwhile, Alice's husband, Roger, was helping Arequipa's patients in another way. A man living across the county road from the sanatorium kept a collection of hunting dogs, which he also trained. The perfect acoustics of the little valley meant that barking, whining, and police whistles disturbed the patients, though after Emma Applegren complained, the owner made some attempts to keep the dogs quiet. But then the hunter sold the property, and it was turned into a kennel, which meant more dogs, more barking, more rattled nerves. It got to the point where the women couldn't rest or even sleep at night.

Multiple polite requests followed by less polite demands did no good, so Applegren asked Roger Kent to step in. He wrote letters to the kennel's owners and said he was going to take legal action if they didn't keep the dogs quiet, but nothing changed. In the late fall of 1951 he filed suit against the kennel. The following spring he took depositions from staff and patients about how the barking affected their work or their recovery. He told everyone to keep detailed diaries of how much barking they heard and for how long. The case was settled out of court, and peace was eventually restored.[2]

Two months after A Night in Peru, a Marin County woman named Bernice Swigard suggested that the party committee formally organize to plan other benefits for Arequipa. In November 1951, Swigard, Kent, and more than twenty other women met for lunch and held the first meeting of a group they named Friends of Arequipa.

By the end of the year, the money they had raised paid for a larger kitchen storeroom and more dressing rooms for up patients. The sanatorium also needed new plumbing and foundation work, which would cost an additional $15,000. So Kent, Swigard, and their dedicated friends began planning the next fund-raiser, to be held in June 1952: A Night in Hawaii.[3]

∽

As all this planning and legal action was going on, the number of patients in Arequipa's beds was dropping. Tuberculosis was still a threat, but many doctors were now giving women isoniazid to take at home, so they didn't need to spend time in a sanatorium. Dr. Cabot Brown was slowly being converted to the new way of treating TB, but he was not ready to give up on the rest cure just yet— especially for women he knew personally. One of them was named Bonnie (a pseudonym).

She found out she had TB in a very roundabout way. Bonnie lived in the YWCA Residence Club in San Francisco, on the Powell Street cable car line. One day she decided to give blood at a local blood bank. She was so thin that the staff turned her down, but they decided to give her a chest X-ray anyway, which was a regular procedure at some facilities. About a month later she got a letter saying she had something on her lung and that she should see her doctor. She threw the paper in the trash, thinking it was nothing to worry about. Then she got a very bad cold and had trouble getting her strength back. A second notice about her lung came in the mail, and she finally decided to do something about it.

Dr. Cabot Brown was a friend of her mother's, and Bonnie called his office to get an appointment. He took another set of X-rays and then told her to sit in the waiting room until the last patient was gone at the end of the workday. Dr. Brown then locked the door, sat down next to Bonnie, and told her she had TB. She was appalled, but when she thought about it, she was really not too shocked, considering how bad she had been feeling. Brown asked her if she had any money and she said no, but after the doctor spoke with her mother and arranged for her to help with the bills, he sent Bonnie to Arequipa in December 1951.

She was still in the early stage, so Dr. Brown put her in the Wing, where the up patients were. He said it would be good for her morale to be around active and cheerful women, but all the other patients went to the dining room for meals, and she had to stay behind and eat off a tray in her bed. That made her depressed. Sometimes a cleaning woman came into the Wing when most other patients were away from the ward and flung her dust mop around while she talked to Bonnie, which didn't make the food any more appetizing.

The Wing was still screened, though the other two wards had been enclosed with glass by this time. Medical treatments and drugs were replacing the all-air-all-the-time philosophy, however slowly. Since it was winter, Bonnie had an electric blanket, and she wore a sweater, a bathrobe, and a stocking cap. She was allowed to read, do crossword puzzles, and knit in bed; she usually read so she could keep one hand warm under the covers. The up patients also came by to talk to her, and just watching their activities around the ward was entertaining.

Cabot Brown didn't give Bonnie any medications but did give her regular X-rays, time in front of the fluoroscope, and a treatment called pneumoperi-toneum, which she loathed. This was an injection of nitrogen or oxygen into the abdominal area to literally lift the lungs from underneath, putting them at rest. Not only did it blow up her abdomen, but it gave her a lot of pain in the shoulders, though once she was back in bed, the pain went away quickly.

Drs. Lloyd Dickey and Glenroy Pierce took care of the everyday situations at Arequipa, but Cabot Brown came by at least once a week to check on everyone. Bonnie liked Dr. Pierce but felt more comfortable with Dr. Dickey. She was only in her twenties, and the more fatherly, older man gave her more confidence. But she preferred Cabot Brown over all of them. He was a giant, handsome, with a shock of white hair even though he was not yet fifty, another genetic legacy from his grandmother. He was dignified but had a twinkle in his eye and that great sense of humor that Lois Downey enjoyed twenty years earlier. He was implacable about defeating TB though, and some of the patients were a little scared of him.

Bonnie was able to go home after just four months in Arequipa, though Cabot Brown still wanted to keep an eye on her. He said she could work in his office in the mornings but only on the condition that she went home in the afternoons and went straight to bed to rest.

About a month before Bonnie left Arequipa, someone in the ward passed around the latest issue of *Life* magazine. One of its articles was titled "TB Milestone: Two New Drugs Give Real Hope of Defeating the Dread Disease." Although it wasn't named, the story was about isoniazid—how it was more powerful than streptomycin and didn't have some of its side effects. In typical *Life* manner, the article was short and succinct, covering only two pages, but it was illustrated with eight photographs. One of them showed a group of women at New York's Sea View Hospital dressed in street clothes and bathrobes with the caption, "Patients dance in a hallway at Sea View Hospital to demonstrate for a newspaper photographer how miraculously the drugs have restored their energy."[4]

The next time Dr. Cabot Brown came to Arequipa, Bonnie showed him the magazine and asked what he thought about the article. He looked at the photos, sniffed, and replied, "Well, if they were my patients, they would dance right back to bed."[5]

Cabot belonged to a number of anti-TB associations, and just like his father he spoke to these groups about medical developments and the state of the sanatorium whenever he could. In April 1953 he was the guest speaker at the annual membership dinner meeting of the Marin County Tuberculosis Association. This wasn't just a self-congratulatory get-together; any resident of Marin County who had bought Christmas Seals the previous year was invited to eat with the doctors.

In March of that year Cabot and his wife, Peggy, went to Tacoma, Washington, and watched with pride as their oldest son was married. A few weeks later they boarded a liner headed for Europe and spent the next two years living in Paris. Official records and family lore are fuzzy about just what Cabot was doing, but his work involved improving the health of postwar residents and refugees. He worried about the increase in tuberculosis in Europe, and he asked his colleagues in the States to send him Christmas Seals, which he sold in France to raise TB awareness. He asked Dr. Pierce to run Arequipa while he was gone and told him to rely on Emma Applegren to manage daily matters as she always had.[6]

∽

The Friends of Arequipa kept up with its work when Cabot was out of the country, of course. It was an independent organization that ran with his blessing, not his involvement. A Night in Hawaii was as successful a fund-raiser as A Night in Peru, and the Friends knew this winning formula would keep money flowing to the sanatorium. After the A Night in Old Vienna gala in September 1953, Arequipa's interior was repainted a soft gray-green, the rattan furniture was sprayed the same color, and the cushions were recovered in greens and corals. New light fixtures were installed, and a new French door now led to the outdoor tiled terrace. By the end of the year, the Friends of Arequipa had raised $33,050.52—enough money to renovate the kitchen with new cabinets and Formica countertops, new appliances, and updated plumbing.[7]

The group was so large that the women formed individual units to take on smaller projects that were just as important as new construction. In February 1954 the Friends established a fund to help women pay for their medical treatment, and Emma Applegren was in charge of how the money was spent. The following May, a group of Friends organized a Motor Corps. Some women took outpatient treatment at Arequipa, such as drug therapy and pneumoperitoneum, and the Friends used their own cars to pick the patients up at home and take them to Arequipa. Another unit went on personal shopping trips for the patients at local stores.

The patients knew what Marin County's women were doing for them. They were grateful and wrote a letter to the editor of the *Daily Independent-Journal* to say what was on their minds: "We wish to express our appreciation to the 'Friends of Arequipa' for the interest they have shown in making our stay in the sanatorium more pleasant—especially for the many extra favors such as the monthly shopping, providing reading material, etc., also the monthly parties in which the trays are attractively arranged with favors, fancy place mats and baskets of candy, also a surprise in some sort of food." The letter was signed "The Girls of Arequipa."[8]

In the summer of 1954 the Friends' husbands threw a barbecue at Arequipa, grilling chicken in the wards while a local high school senior named Betsy played guitar and sang cowboy songs. The children in residence remembered when she had come by the previous December to sing them Christmas carols, and in spite of the hot July evening, they asked her to play "Jingle Bells" and other snowy favorites. Betsy came back during Christmas of 1955 to sing at the Friends' holiday party, which was now an annual tradition.

Cabot Brown and his wife returned to the United States in August 1955, and he was soon confronted with some serious financial problems at Arequipa. Admissions had been dropping, thanks to improvements in the antibiotics doctors could use, which meant less income. Someone (either Dr. Pierce or Emma Applegren) had not paid some unemployment taxes for the nurses, so a tax bill was also due.[9]

Help came four months later in the form of a Ford Foundation grant. The foundation gave money to a variety of organizations in northern California in December 1955, and Arequipa's piece of the pie was $18,700, which is equal to about $174,000 today. The money was likely put into the sanatorium itself and not sent to the IRS.[10]

The Friends of Arequipa were still busy with their own fund-raising, and they continued to rely on Emma Applegren to let them know what was needed and to manage how the funds were spent. But in 1955, after twenty years as Arequipa's superintendent, she decided it was time to retire. This was a blow to everyone, but Applegren was now in her early sixties and had things she wanted to do. Within weeks she was succeeded by Gertrude Hickey, originally from Reno, Nevada, where she had worked as a laboratory technician, though she was also a nurse. She got into the routine quickly, and the Friends brought her into their circle right away.[11]

When massive storms caused flooding and damage at Arequipa in early 1956, the Friends hosted a Leap Year Dance to raise money to make repairs. The individual units were now as busy as the larger organization, and the women regularly brought hairdressers to the sanatorium for beauty days and held fashion shows as fund-raisers.[12]

When 1956 opened, Cabot did something that would have shocked his father: he decided to admit male patients to Arequipa. This move wasn't a general call for male consumptives but rather an attempt to bring more income into the sanatorium. The county physician for Marin, Dr. Rafael Dufficy, had asked local hospitals to place bids on providing beds and care for low-income male TB patients; the county would pay the cost for their care. Cabot Brown put in a bid but was outraged when Dr. Dufficy addressed the board of supervisors at a meeting and told them that Arequipa was not equipped to take men into its wards. The women-only policy was the problem; Dr. Dufficy thought that Arequipa could not be converted quickly enough to admit men; nor could it accept advanced-stage cases.

At the meeting Cabot did not hide his anger. He told the supervisors that these statements were just not true and noted that he had put in a lower bid than Ross Hospital, which eventually won the contract. But there was nothing he could do. County officials said they would review his proposal again, but they stuck with their original decision.

Why Cabot took such a desperate step to keep Arequipa financially sound is understandable, but it would have been complicated. With only around twenty or twenty-five patients on hand at a time, it would have been easy to devote separate wards to men and women, something that was impossible when the sanatorium fairly bulged with sick women and every bed was full. Life would not have been the same for his staff though.

The male doctors would have taken the change in stride, but the nurses, some of whom had been at Arequipa for many years, might have found caring for male patients difficult. The day-to-day treatment would the same, but they could be on the receiving end of everything from flirtation to harassment. Arequipa's nurses were autonomous and highly trained, and they often made medical decisions when the doctors were not available.

This ran counter to attitudes about the role of women in medicine, which had progressed, but not too far. Stereotypes about nurses ranged from glorified cleaning lady to sex object, the latter being predominant thanks to World War II pin-up images and the proliferation of "sexy nurse" postcards in the following decade.[13] But the nurses never had to face this cultural change.

Cabot did not enter a bid with the county to take male patients in 1957 because a rumor was bubbling underneath the changes in personnel, the shopping, the medical treatments, the interagency squabbling, and the daily routine. It ran around the wards, at Friends' lunches, and in doctors' offices: Arequipa was going to close.

~

It began in the spring of 1957, when admissions took a steep decline. There were now only fifteen to eighteen patients in residence at a time, instead of the usual forty. Local reporters asked Dr. Cabot Brown about the rumor, but he denied it, saying that yes, fewer women sought treatment, but they still needed Arequipa's help. He knew the sanatorium would close someday, because drugs were no longer something experimental. They were part of a doctor's anti-TB arsenal. But not everyone responded to the drugs, and the rest cure was still essential for women who had no other recourse. It was also still affordable, something else that Cabot Brown had never changed. He thought Arequipa might have three more years of usefulness.

Departures from the wards increased, and admissions slowed even further through the early summer of 1957; only five women lived in the wards around Independence Day. Dr. Cabot Brown, as much a realist as his father, took stock and made the only decision he could, despite his optimistic outlook. He announced that Arequipa would close on August 1.

He had always planned that when the inevitable happened, he would turn the sanatorium over to an organization or institution that had similar ideals. He thought perhaps the building could be converted into a polio hospital, but in the end, he found the Marin County chapter of the Society for Crippled Children and Adults. This group created programs of recreation and rehabilitation for the disabled, and both the building and the beautiful setting were perfect for the work it hoped to do. The society leased the property from the Arequipa Foundation, which had superseded the Bothin Convalescent Home as the corporate entity with oversight over the sanatorium.[14]

Throughout August, Dr. Brown arranged for the remaining patients to get outpatient treatment or a bed at another sanatorium in the Bay Area. The nurses, Gertrude Hickey, and the housekeeping staff trickled away to other jobs as soon as the patients were gone. On September 1, 1957, the Society for Crippled Children and Adults started moving its people in. The sanatorium was renamed the Arequipa Center.

The Society for Crippled Children and Adults got something else in the deal. Without skipping a beat, the Friends of Arequipa turned their fund-raising efforts toward the needs of the society. By December they were already planning a New Year's Eve benefit.[15]

Arequipa was so much a part of Marin's history that its closing received a lot of press coverage. The same thing happened in the medical literature. The January 1958 issue of the *Bulletin of the Marin County Medical Society* published a long article about Arequipa's history and its new owners. Written by prominent Marin County doctor and amateur naturalist Robert West, the piece included a short section about the Friends of Arequipa and how the women had voted unanimously to support the disabled.

Arequipa the place of rest was now in the past, Dr. West wrote. But it had a bright future providing services to people who most needed them, which was wholly in the spirit of its founder, Dr. Philip King Brown. "The good that men do," he concluded, "is not always interred with their bones."[16]

The Society for Crippled Children and Adults gave up its lease on the Arequipa property at the end of 1959, and a new tenant was already interested. By June 1960 the regional Girl Scout Council had completed negotiations to take over the land and the buildings for its local troops.

Corena Green was a reporter for the *Daily Independent-Journal* when all these changes were happening at Arequipa. She was a tireless Marin County volunteer for causes ranging from the Red Cross to orphaned children to the American Association of University Women. She was also a former president of the Marin County Girl Scout Council and a fixture of its publicity committee. When the Scouts made their announcement about Arequipa, Green wrote a long newspaper article about the sanatorium and the Girl Scouts' plans for the property. She also included a plea for donations to help fund some needed restoration and rebuilding.

But she saw something in this story beyond a simple real estate transaction and stated it right up front with the title of her article: "Marin County Girl Scouts Adopt Arequipa Aims with Acquisition." While most people saw Arequipa as an old sanatorium that had passed into history, Corena Green saw it as something intangible but strong—a force that lifted women out of fear and illness, and still had the power to change women's lives.

She put it this way. "So 50 years later the profile of Arequipa changes but not the heart nor the intent. The early pioneers and patients returning now surely would see only progress in the program about to be launched at the site—a program designed to produce happy, healthy young women, ready to take their place in the American scene."[17]

⌇

When antibiotics made the rest cure obsolete, old sanatorium buildings—crumbling, scarred, and sad—were transformed, some by demolition and obliteration, others by renovation or a personality change.

Many sanatoria were turned into hospitals or clinics and, depending on their management, were proud of their early history as places where people were treated for TB. The Barlow Sanatorium in Los Angeles, now the Barlow Respiratory Hospital, is one example. Its founding as a sanatorium more than a century ago by Dr. W. Jarvis Barlow is an important part of its story. The entire town of Saranac Lake, New York, was dedicated to TB treatment when Dr. Edward Trudeau established his first sanatorium there, and today Historic Saranac Lake preserves its buildings and its story with events and education.

These are the success stories, but they are rare. Sanatoria were, and in some cases still are, unnerving places. This is especially true for those whose original function is misunderstood or forgotten. Although tuberculosis is still around and is increasing in some populations, most people who live near former sanatoria have never known anyone with TB. Some of the buildings are derelict and unused but not yet torn down, and this is how weird reputations are formed and spread.

Ghost-hunting groups and television shows like *Ghost Adventures* regularly visit decrepit former TB sanatoria, such as Waverly Hills Sanatorium in Kentucky, San Haven in North Dakota, and the Lima Tuberculosis Hospital in Ohio. There, the spirits of mistreated patients are said to loom like malevolent shadows. Locals talk up the creepy history of nearby sanatoria. A crumbling, unused building, where people once had a disease that no one has ever experienced, must surely be haunted.

Arequipa, however, escaped this fate. The Girl Scouts kept up the old hospital building, which they named Brown House, and used it for gatherings and sleepovers for decades. When Happy Stanton took over as site manager in the early 1980s, the building was beginning to crumble a little, though it was still useful. But in 1984 Arequipa succumbed to the weight of its own long history.

Years of heavy rains had eroded the soil around the foundation, and despite surviving a major earthquake in 1957, the building was far from seismically safe. In the fall of 1984, the graceful shingled building was torn down, leaving only the cement substructure behind. The Girl Scout Council had improved the property enough that it could still hold yearly encampments there. It also used the buildings at the former Hill Farm property, now called the Bothin Youth Center. But something of the sanatorium still lingered, and it exerted an intangible influence on the people closest to it.

Happy and his wife, Cari Lyn, lived in Ashe House, a rambling bungalow on the Bothin Youth Center side of the hill, built around 1910 for Elizabeth Ashe herself. The upper level of the long, two-story house held three bedrooms. The largest, the master bedroom, had rickety screened windows on three sides that went all the way to the ceiling.

In August 1987, on the day of her thirty-fifth birthday, Cari Lyn suffered the rupture of a tubal or ectopic pregnancy for the second time in her life. Rushed to a local hospital, suffering massive internal bleeding, she was pulled back from death and sent home to recover. Ten days later she had a third rupture, causing more bleeding, and in her already weakened state she collapsed unconscious in her bathroom. Happy called for an ambulance once again, and Cari Lyn woke up in the hospital, alive but physically and emotionally crushed.

Blood was on everyone's mind in 1987. The AIDS epidemic made transfusions questionable, if not dangerous, and even though supplies were now being screened, some doctors were reluctant to give blood except under the most dire of circumstances. Cari Lyn's condition was not considered dire enough, though even without a transfusion she got hepatitis during her hospital stay. Once she was stable, the doctors sent her home and said that rest was what she needed for her recovery and to allow her body to rebuild its own blood.

Back at Ashe House, Happy helped Cari Lyn up the stairs to their bedroom and into bed. Its head was on the eastern, screened wall of the house, and while under the covers, propped on pillows, Cari Lyn could just see out the windows, where her view took in the northern and western portions of the little glen that held their home. And there she stayed for the next twelve months.

She slept twenty hours a day for weeks, and when she had the strength and the appetite, she craved foods such as liver, red cabbage, beef, beans, and tomatoes. Happy fixed her whatever she wanted, whenever she needed it. Raised a Christian Scientist, Cari Lyn knew how to listen to her body and understood its needs. What she didn't know at the time was that she had chosen to live like a TB patient.

Rest is a relative term today, and when doctors prescribe it, they aren't exactly specific about what it means. To tuberculosis physicians like Philip King Brown, Ethel Owen, Mary Jones Mentzer, and Cabot Brown, the word came with a list of things that patients could and could not do. Cari Lyn also knew how to define it for herself, and without intention, her experience mirrored the lives of the women who had breathed the scented air in the next valley over so many years before.

She lived high above the world, and with her head to the east, she watched the sun's progression and the movement of the stars through windows that she and Happy kept open all year round. The borders of her life were screens, and the substance of her breath was the unobstructed air scented with bay, oak, and fragrant Scotch broom. In autumn the fogs tumbled into her room, making her furniture look ghostly.

It was quiet in her valley, though the kennel that still operated across the road from the old sanatorium boarded dogs, whose barking sometimes rent the night air. When the Girl Scouts held their camps at the Arequipa property, the songs they sang around the campfire at night echoed all the way to Ashe House, sweet voices lulling her to sleep. Not everything was peaceful, though. Nightmares plagued her, and for months she remembered only their awful images and not her waking hours.

By the spring of 1988, the light began to come back into Cari Lyn's life, and she was able to get up and walk around a little bit each day. She felt like she was walking through water and she did her own version of the TB glide around the house until her strength came back. Cari Lyn was more aware of what was going on around her and realized that it was the silence and peace of the place that brought her back to life and sanity.

The disruption of her life, and almost its loss, had transformed her into a new person, and all unknowing, she had followed Dr. Philip King Brown's prescription. Within the space of another year she was fully healed, and she and Happy, now truly living up to his name because his wife was still with him, soon moved to a new city for the next phase of their lives.[18]

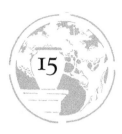

AFTERLIVES

NO ONE WHO WAS EITHER TREATED at Arequipa or worked there left the sanatorium unchanged. For the doctors and nurses, work at the sanatorium was personally and professionally fulfilling and was a stepping stone for long careers—especially for the women.

Dr. Emma Willits continued to practice at Children's Hospital during the years she worked as a visiting physician at Arequipa and afterward. She also became a renowned surgeon. Dr. Willits retired in 1934 and in 1941 was honored for her service at a reception at Children's Hospital. She would not accept a personal gift, so the hospital bought a new operating table in her name. The *San Francisco Chronicle* described the scene: "For years she wore sterile white and a mask as she approached the operating table. But yesterday, between the hours of 4 and 6 o'clock the slim, gray-haired Dr. Willits was a debutante, not the dean of women surgeons in San Francisco." She was honored again in 1951 during the groundbreaking for the hospital's new building, and she died there in April 1965 at the age of ninety-five. She directed that her body be buried in her hometown of Macedon, New York.[1]

Dr. Mary Mentzer, who held Arequipa together when Dr. Philip King Brown was serving in France during World War I, spent the rest of her life quietly practicing medicine from her office on Hyde Street, just a few doors down the hall from Dr. Cabot Brown. She was also on the board of the San Francisco County Medical Society. She passed away in 1955 at the age of seventy-seven.[2]

Dr. Ethel Owen continued to work as a public health physician and surgeon after she left Arequipa. She was on the board of directors of the Women's City Club and the National League for Women's Service throughout the 1940s, and in 1944 the nursing school at her alma mater, Stanford University, gave a tea to commemorate her long career. She retired soon after, but Ethel Owen was one of those women for whom retirement simply means being busy doing something different.

She loved to travel, and throughout the 1950s and early 1960s she went to Europe, the Panama Canal Zone, and the Caribbean. She especially loved to visit Panama, perhaps remembering when she heard President Theodore Roosevelt speak about the canal when she was a young Stanford student. She moved to Aptos, on the peninsula south of San Francisco, and gave talks about her travels to women's groups like the American Association of University Women. She was also an avid reader of Shakespeare and led book club discussions of his plays. She kept up this schedule almost to the day of her death at seventy-nine in December 1969.[3]

The male doctors Cabot Brown hired and who gave the most time to Arequipa continued with their already successful careers after their sanatorium service. Pediatrician Lloyd Dickey continued his work with tubercular children and joined a medical organization that is today Kaiser Permanente. He died in 1974. Dr. Glenroy Pierce left California for the Oregon State Tuberculosis Hospital and in 1960 became medical superintendent of the Arkansas Tuberculosis Sanatorium in Booneville, dying suddenly at the age of fifty in 1961. Dr. Harry J. Pruett died at age sixty-five in 1956 at his home in San Francisco's fashionable Russian Hill district. Ten years earlier a judge had denied his wife, Alberta, a divorce, saying that her husband rising at 6:30 A.M. to get Popsicles for their children did not constitute cruelty. They stayed married until the doctor's death.[4]

Dr. Thomas Wiper, Rose's favorite (next to Cabot Brown), had lived in the Marin County bay-side town of Sausalito since 1937, but he lived in Burlingame when he was in charge of the nearby California Sanatorium in Belmont. He retired to his Marin home in 1967, and though he and Rose did not stay in touch, she and her husband tried to visit Dr. Wiper when they learned he was suffering from dementia in the early 1970s. Though his wife, Sybil, was touched by their concern, she wouldn't let Rose see her former mentor because she wanted the young woman to remember him as he had been. He died in 1974 at the age of seventy.[5]

For reasons lost to history, nurse Elizabeth MacMillan never had another job after she left Arequipa. She may have been ill; she gave up her position there around 1940, when she was in her mid-sixties, and died in 1945. She still lived in San Anselmo, the little town down the road from Arequipa. It was her wish to be cremated and to have her ashes placed with those of her brother, who had lived in southern California for many years and was interred in a cemetery in Compton.[6]

~

The other staff members who braved weather, trains, and lurching ferry rides to treat Arequipa's patients all profited from their time there and took these lessons into their own afterlives, especially those who continued with TB work. Dr. Anna Davenport, for example, was Arequipa's first radiologist; her next job mirrored her position at Arequipa almost exactly.

Around 1917 she moved to New York, living part-time in the little town of Santa Clara, just a few miles from Saranac Lake. During the summers she was the resident physician for the Vacation Home for Working Girls in Santa Clara, which housed young women in two buildings, called Hill Crest and Uplands. The Working Girls' Vacation Society, which oversaw the properties, had been founded in 1885 by George E. Dodge, a lumber millionaire. After his death, his widow made an endowment on the Santa Clara homes to keep them in business. Like Arequipa, Hill Crest and Uplands offered affordable tuberculosis care to working women and girls in a beautiful setting and taught them how to keep TB at bay after they went home.

When she wasn't in Santa Clara, Dr. Davenport lived in Hartford, Connecticut, where she had lived before interning in Boston and California. She was a mainstay of the Hartford Dispensary, a clinic founded in 1871 that was much like Dr. Charlotte Brown's first dispensary in San Francisco. It served members of the community who couldn't afford to go to a private doctor, and she was a board member there for decades. She was also a staunch temperance advocate and belonged to the local chapter of the Woman's Christian Temperance Union. She gave talks at many of its meetings and spoke about the medical dangers of drink, leaving the moral issue to others. Dr. Davenport retired from her work at the dispensary in 1947, when she was in her mid-seventies, and died the following year.[7]

Lucy Pyle, trained as a nurse but who had spent her time at Arequipa as a social worker, found her next calling working with children at risk for TB. She left Arequipa in 1920 and immediately went to work as superintendent of the San Mateo Preventorium. She was there for about two years, and, after some time off in Hawaii, she gave her skills and experience to two other preventoriums in southern California: Rest Haven in San Diego and El Nido in Pasadena. She was also a member of the California Tuberculosis Association and gave a paper at its Los Angeles meeting in 1925.

The Bay Area beckoned again, and in 1926 Lucy Pyle moved to Berkeley, where she worked as a nurse inspector for the Berkeley school system. She spent the next four years watching over children's lungs and doing public health nursing. In 1930, at the age of fifty-two, she moved back home to Siskiyou County in far northern California, where she lived with her sister-in-law and worked as a public health nurse in the ranching town of Table Rock. She then married Charles Hast, retired, and passed away in 1956 at seventy-eight years old.[8]

∽

The women who ran Arequipa's day-to-day operations as superintendents came to their jobs with multiple skills and had varying post-sanatorium lives. Nora Harnden, after retreating to Europe when she left Arequipa under a cloud, came back to California and immediately went the other direction, to Hawaii, where her brother was a U.S. consul. In the early 1920s she lived in Oakland and Alameda, and was very involved with the Business Women's Club. By 1930 she was living in Carmel, on the Monterey Peninsula. She traveled again to Europe and was back in the Bay Area by the early 1950s. She doesn't seem to have continued with her nursing or taken another job, and perhaps she did not have a financial need to do so. She died in 1957, aged eighty-six.[9]

Ethel Steeves, nurse and superintendent, visited family members in Seattle in 1930, soon after leaving Arequipa, then returned to the Bay Area to continue her nursing career in both San Francisco and the East Bay cities of Berkeley and Alameda, though it's not known when she retired. She died in October 1965, at eighty-seven years old.[10]

Eva Gregg took her passion for remodeling and redecorating into the position she accepted a year after leaving Arequipa: director of the Girls' Friendly Society Lodge in San Francisco, just a few blocks from the downtown district. This was a type of residential hotel, a safe place for young women to live, complete with baths and kitchens as well as reception rooms and a big dining room. Soon after taking over as director, Gregg overhauled the slightly shabby building, much as she had done for Arequipa in 1932. (The building is now the Queen Anne Hotel.) She continued to lecture around the Bay Area about her years as missionary in China. She retired and moved to Berkeley in the early 1950s and died at seventy in 1956.[11]

After twenty years as Arequipa's superintendent, Emma Applegren left Marin County and two years later married a man in Monterey named Oscar Carlson. They moved to the town of Vista, north of San Diego. There, Emma gardened and wrote long letters to the nurses she had met while studying at Northwestern and those she served with in France during World War I. Having a nursing career and facing an enemy overseas had bonded the women together, a phenomenon not exclusive to male soldiers. Emma attended reunions at Northwestern when she could and was still writing to her colleagues in the early 1970s when she entered her eighth decade.[12]

～

Many benefactors and volunteers continued to fight TB in their own ways.

Mary Holton and her husband, Luther, who were among Arequipa's original funders, moved to Toronto around 1920. (Luther Holton was a Canadian native.) Mary took on the role of treasurer for the Ladies' Auxiliary Board of the Hamilton Health Association, which operated the Mountain Sanatorium and treated TB patients from all over the province of Ontario. The Holtons stayed in Canada for the rest of their lives, and Mary continued to volunteer for the sanatorium. She died in 1935, at the age of sixty-eight, a few years after her husband's death.[13]

Elsie Krafft started volunteering at Arequipa in 1915 as a secretary and social worker and more than thirty years later was still offering counsel to the patients there. She also worked for many other medical and charitable organizations in the Bay Area, from the Child Guidance Clinic to the Community Chest, and kept an office in Dr. Cabot Brown's medical suite in downtown San Francisco. She lived in the Krafft family home until a few years before her death, when she moved into the Women's City Club near San Francisco's Union Square. She was a wealthy woman, thanks to the legacy of her father's successful architectural career.

She died in October 1962, at the age of eighty-seven, and left a sizable chunk of her estate to Arequipa. With the sanatorium now closed, Dr. Cabot Brown, whom Krafft designated to manage the bequest, had to find a good use for the funds. He used the gift to endow a laboratory in Palo Alto, which stayed in business for decades.[14]

Jeannette Jordan did not live to see Arequipa flourish like most of her sister benefactors did. She died in 1920, and when her will was read, Dr. Philip Brown was astonished to learn that she had left Arequipa $25,000. She was very specific about how her bequest was to be used: "To Doctor Philip King Brown and S. I. Wormser, and to the survivor as trustees, I give the sum of $25,000, in trust, to be used by them in said way they think best to further and carry out the objects for which the Arequipa Sanitorium at Fairfax, Marin County, California, is created, but to be used solely and exclusively, for said Sanitorium."

Dr. Brown wrote about this gift in the annual report that came out after Jordan's death. He called it the Jordan Bequest, and though the words he used to acknowledge Jordan seem a little stilted today, they were no doubt deeply heartfelt. The bequest, he said, was "one of the examples of thoughtful help which so characterized her interest."[15]

Elizabeth Ashe, the founder of Hill Farm, the convalescent home for children just over the hill from Arequipa, was a powerful presence as the sanatorium was being conceived and built. She was on the board of directors for many years, but once Arequipa was up and running, she turned her attention to the Telegraph Hill Neighborhood House, her settlement house in San Francisco and, of course, the continuing work at Hill Farm. After running the Red Cross Children's Bureau in France during World War I, she came back to San Francisco and jumped into more social service work.

She supported Prohibition, knowing how drunkenness plagued the women and children of Telegraph Hill. She championed the expansion of a visiting nurse service, spoke out for children who were being pulled into "delinquency," and also supported the work of her partner, Alice Griffith, in her advocacy for decent housing for the poor. Elizabeth Ashe was named an honorary consultant to the San Francisco Department of Public Health when she was seventy years old, and the last years of her life were devoted to the construction of a modern building for her settlement house. She died in January 1954 at age eighty-five, and her obituaries and the real mourning that enveloped the city of San Francisco were a tribute to her influence and the impact she had on the Bay Area. The Telegraph Hill Neighborhood Center still serves the people of North Beach.[16]

Henry Bothin died in 1923, leaving behind the legacies of both Hill Farm and Arequipa, as well as the Bothin Helping Fund, which he established in 1917. Organized to support these two Marin County organizations, it expanded its mission after the death of the founder and namesake and is now the Bothin Foundation. The foundation grants approximately $2 million every year to Bay Area nonprofits, encompassing everything from arts organizations to groups that work with disadvantaged children.[17]

∽

But of course, all these men and women came to Arequipa for one reason: the patients. Most of them walked away to hopeful new lives, free of lung disease, but tuberculosis always lurked, like a relative no one ever invites to family reunions. And sometimes the rest cure only went so far, only giving a few months' respite before the inevitable. But the women who took Philip and Cabot Brown's teachings, lectures, and training home with them had the best chance for life, for a truce with their scarred lungs.

Patty is an example. When she decided to leave Arequipa in May 1950, Dr. Cabot Brown gave her some very strict rules to follow at home. She had to use different dishes and silverware from the rest of her family. She couldn't kiss her children or taste their food, and she had to stand at least an arm's distance away from people when she was talking to them. Dr. Brown also said she needed outpatient treatment, and for nearly four more years, Patty took streptomycin and came back to Arequipa regularly to get the pneumoperitoneum treatment. It made her look six months pregnant all the time, but it was better than lying in bed in a sanatorium, looking out the window.

After she got home, Patty noticed that many of her friends avoided her like poison. This was hard, but standing aloof from her children was harder. She decided that the only way to change this was to make sure she got healthy and stayed that way. She started to do a bit more physical labor around her house, watched her health, took her medicine religiously, and began to put a toe into her former social life.

It didn't take long for her confidence to come back and for friends to see that she wasn't Typhoid Mary. She soon embraced her children again and had two more girls, and as the years went by, she never had a relapse. Patty got involved with Marin County politics and was a fixture in her neighborhood for her activism. She died in 2017 at the age of ninety-four.[18]

Bonnie had a rougher time after she departed Arequipa in 1952. She worked in Dr. Cabot Brown's office for a while and followed his advice about resting in the afternoon. But she defied him in another way: she had been a smoker before going into Arequipa and started up again once she went home. When Cabot Brown found out she was smoking, he backed her into the fluoroscopy room in his office and gave her a lecture that made her feel about two inches tall. She knew why he had to talk to her the way he did. He was fighting TB in his own way, even if he had to bully a woman to do it. (Ironically, Cabot Brown himself was a longtime chain-smoker.)

In 1955 Bonnie's health broke down and she had to spend seven months in a tuberculosis sanatorium in the northern mountain town of Redding, California, where she later gave birth to a daughter. But she pulled herself and her health together and twenty-five years later moved back to Marin County, still on her feet. She died in 2004 at seventy-seven years old.[19]

The occupational skills that Rose learned at Arequipa sent her fully prepared into the rest of her working life. She spent three years with Dr. Wiper at the California Sanatorium in Belmont, doing clerical and laboratory work, but she was never satisfied with the knowledge she already had. Years of lying in bed had made her mind run to ambition, rather than invalidism, so to make sure she was keeping up with whatever tasks Dr. Wiper might set, she took a course in medical stenography. She never needed it, but she was ready just in case.

Rose often visited one of her sisters in San Francisco on the weekends, taking a taxi to the main road in Belmont and then a bus into the city. On Sunday nights she would wait alone in a rather seedy part of downtown San Francisco, where a few of the male Filipino workers at the sanatorium would pick her up and take her back to her job at Belmont.

In 1950 a friend persuaded Rose to take the U.S. Civil Service exam. She didn't have a high school diploma, but she was still allowed to sit for the test. She passed it handily and took a job with the U.S. Army in the procurement division at San Francisco's Fort Mason, later transferring to the Oakland Army Base during the Korean War.

Rose got married in 1951. Gertrude, the woman who had laced her orange juice with wheat germ at Arequipa, also kept her health after leaving the sanatorium and started a catering business. The two women remained friends, and Gertrude catered Rose's wedding as her gift to the couple. Rose also stayed close to Emma Applegren, and she and her husband visited Emma after she left Arequipa and was married.

Rose moved up in government service, taking on positions of more responsibility. She decided to get her GED in 1975 because the work world was changing; she didn't want to be left behind because TB had kept her from going to high school. It was a good move; the following year she landed a job with the Small Business Administration.

Her husband died in 1978, and after a visit to Washington, D.C., with a sister-in-law the following year, Rose decided to upend her life and move across the country. The main office of the Small Business Administration hired her in D.C., and she stayed for three years. She worked on and off at Garfinckel's department store, where she became the personal shopper for some of Washington's most influential women, including Supreme Court justice Sandra Day O'Connor, with whom she once shared a Coke. One of her coworkers was the mother of *Washington Post* reporter Carl Bernstein. Rose also assisted the wives of diplomats and visiting dignitaries. She remembers one visit most vividly.

One day a collection of men wearing either dark suits or Nehru jackets came onto the sales floor, accompanied by Sonia Gandhi, the daughter-in-law of Indira Gandhi, India's prime minister. She made a number of purchases but was concerned about how well they would be wrapped, so Rose took her to the back room to show her how it was done. They didn't tell Gandhi's FBI and Indian security detail that they were leaving the area, and when the men noticed Sonia was gone, they immediately assumed she had been kidnapped. Luckily, Rose brought her back to the public area before they could mobilize a strike team.

Rose took a break from retail after a couple of years and worked in purchasing at Fort Belvoir in Virginia. She had considerable government experience, so she decided to apply for a management position but was turned down because of her gender. Disgusted, she stayed on as the assistant to the purchasing manager but waited for the day she could retire, which came in the early 1990s.

As she aged, Rose spent time enjoying herself: going to museums, volunteering in the White House during the Bill Clinton administration and for People to People International. She also traveled, visiting cities where a diplomat friend was posted, but she always returned to Italy, her favorite destination. She loved Italian opera and was a big fan of the tenor Luciano Pavarotti. With age came a few health problems, some related to her long-ago TB, but she managed them and managed to keep traveling until her mid-eighties.

Rose credited Arequipa, Dr. Brown, and Dr. Wiper for restoring her health and her chances for life. "They really did a miraculous job," she recalled. "I don't think they expected me to live." She walked out of the sanatorium knowing how to take care of herself and to keep her TB from returning. But she got something else in the bargain, the very thing that Philip King Brown had built Arequipa for: occupational skills that allowed her to go out into the world and be an independent working woman.

Dr. Brown knew that he was returning women to their husbands and families once they left his sanatorium TB-free. But he also understood the value of work in women's lives, whether it was to support themselves and their children or move into one of the professions that were slowly opening to women's participation. He didn't care why they chose the work they did. He just wanted them to be healthy while they did it.[20]

~

Arequipa's final medical director, Dr. Cabot Brown, brought the sanatorium's administration full circle. In its forty-six-year history, it had been built, supervised, visited, and advised by two generations and four members of the Brown family: Philip, the founder; Phoebe, the little girl who played in the pottery;

Adelaide, who made sure the women had safe milk to drink; and Cabot, who succeeded his father and brought Arequipa into the modern age.

Closing Arequipa was a difficult but necessary decision, but Dr. Brown still had plenty of work to keep him busy. He had a thriving practice in San Francisco and was on the board of directors of the California Tuberculosis Association and the National Tuberculosis Association. He traveled around the state giving free TB tests to schoolkids, including in remote locations such as Happy Camp, on the Klamath River nearly four hundred miles northwest of San Francisco. He was also a valued member of the Placer County Health Association, which watched over the citizens of cities and old gold rush towns around Sacramento.

He also added teaching to his repertoire, serving as an associate clinical professor of medicine at the University of California and Presbyterian Medical Center in San Francisco. He dedicated his private practice to public health and tuberculosis control programs. Cabot was also in charge of the Arequipa Foundation, which succeeded Bothin's original organization. In 1963 it donated a storage refrigerator to the Marin Blood Center.

He was a kind and funny grandfather to his six grandchildren and taught them a number of important skills: how to maneuver a rowboat on Lake Tahoe, how to make a good Scotch and soda, and how play cribbage, dominoes, and Parcheesi (described by his granddaughter Charlotte as a contact sport in their family). Cabot was a fiercely competitive card player, especially bridge, and played at San Francisco's Pacific-Union Club on Nob Hill, a social club dating to 1889. He also had a talent that charmed both his family and party guests: he had perfect pitch and could hear a tune just once and then play it on the piano.

By the late 1960s, Cabot was less agile and could no longer play tennis or even get into and out of a boat. The reason was an untreated broken ankle, which he had sustained in April 1951 when a private plane he was piloting made a hard emergency landing near Santa Cruz. Like many doctors, Cabot ignored his own illnesses and injuries, a trait that later came back to haunt him.

His eyesight also began to fail, and even after cataract surgery, he still had trouble seeing. This did not stop him from driving, which horrified his family, and he was almost as terrifying on the road as his aunt Adelaide had been. When he rolled his Plymouth Valiant down the driveway to go to the Pacific-Union Club, he would also roll down the window so he could hear the children on the street as he drove away. A few years later there was a family coup; Cabot gave up his car keys and the Valiant went up for sale.

Cabot sometimes intervened in his grandchildren's lives. Around 1965 or 1966, Cabot and Peggy took ten-year-old Andrew to Europe for three weeks, showing him London, Paris, Berlin, Nuremberg, and Munich (with Cabot playing bridge along the way). Cabot planned the trip while Andrew was still in school, and for a very specific reason. School administrators wanted Andrew to skip a grade, which was abhorrent to his grandfather. He remembered how hard it was to go to college when he was so young, and he didn't want his grandson to go through the same struggles. The European sojourn was just long enough for Andrew to miss important classes and exams, and he advanced to the next grade with his classmates.

Some of the kids were also on the receiving end of stern lectures about the evils of smoking. Cabot's chain-smoking habit eventually led to his death, the irony of which was not lost on his intelligent grandchildren.

Dr. Cabot Brown died in September 1978 at his home in San Francisco, the city where his grandmother Dr. Charlotte Brown had brought her own young family more than a century before. Her legacy survives in more than one hundred descendants, the majority of whom live on the East or West Coasts, the geography that nurtured their extraordinary ancestor.[21]

∾

What did all the people who served at Arequipa—the women especially—have in common? First and most importantly they possessed a singular desire to heal, and they had many paths to that end: as doctor, nurse, social worker, or benefactor. The women who gave their time to Arequipa came into the work via many different roads, and some went on to very unusual lives and careers. At first glance it might seem as though the sanatorium had no effect on them or their post-Arequipa lives at all, but a closer look at someone like Ynés Mexía reveals another story.

She did not have tuberculosis, but she needed medical help after leaving Mexico and moving to the United States. Frail and nervous, she became Dr. Philip King Brown's patient, and he thought the best way for her to move past her suffering was to serve others. She had no training as a social worker other than what she read in books or discussed with the nurses and women like Lucy Pyle, but Dr. Brown called her a social worker and gave her tasks to make her feel she was useful in the world. From teaching basket making to doing follow-up work with discharged patients, Mexía had responsibilities that affected the lives of other women. She took to the work slowly but then with more confidence.

As the pottery work began to wind down after World War I, and occupational therapy in general was also on its way out at Arequipa, Mexía started taking classes in art and photography. She also joined the Sierra Club, going on hikes through the redwoods, which both awed and calmed her. She then took a few classes in botany and her life took a new direction.

After learning as much as she could about plant taxonomy and classification, Mexía started going on plant collecting expeditions, often with only a few locals to help carry her equipment. Between 1925 and 1938 she wandered through sometimes dangerous territory to find little-known botanicals, traveling from Alaska to the tip of South America. She also took photographs, and her specimens and photos live in many museums and botanical collections today. She discovered a new genus of the aster and sunflower family, which was named for her—*Mexianthus mexicana*—in addition to fifty new species of plants. She died at sixty-eight in July 1938, mourned especially deeply by Helen and Philip King Brown.[22]

Ynés Mexía's life is a perfect example of how places like Arequipa served not only the ill, who were there to be healed, but also those who were doing the healing. Arequipa helped Ynés find emotional and physical strength as she helped women who were worse off than she was. Surrounded by oak and bay trees in Arequipa's quiet glen, she found herself drawn to nature, and it was there that she found the peace she was looking for.

∼

Arequipa still lives today in a beautiful and tangible form: the pottery and tile.

Arequipa bowls, vases, tiles, and tabletops have been discovered and rediscovered by collectors and historians more than once since Dr. Brown closed down the pottery works. The pieces are appealing on so many levels: as examples of California's Arts and Crafts period, as folk art, as a prime example of ceramics as occupational therapy, and as an expression of the place of women in the American art pottery movement.

All of Arequipa's pottery directors went on to stellar careers after they left the sanatorium. After leaving Arequipa, Frederick Rhead opened his own ceramics firm, which lasted until 1917. He spent the rest of his career at commercial ceramic companies. After leaving his teaching job, Albert Solon founded Solon & Schemmel, a tile-making firm called in San Jose. Fred Wilde moved to southern California to work with the Pomona Tile Manufacturing Company, where he stayed until retirement.[23]

Philip King Brown never liked to see anything go to waste. In 1930 he wrote a letter to Albert Solon, asking if he would like to buy some of the old tile molds in storage at Arequipa. Solon told him they weren't really worth saving and in his reply said, "There is no more market for old tiles than for diseased tonsils. . . . Old moulds, unlike old wine find few purchasers."[24]

The pottery the three directors helped create tell Arequipa's story just as well as the annual reports and photographs that Happy Stanton found languishing in the old building. Some vases are simple. They are well formed and solid, but with no carving, just a glaze that might be a bit runny or lumpy. Wide bowls are well carved, but their bottoms are sometimes wobbly. Other pieces are spectacular—intricately molded, carved with surgical precision, glazed with exquisite colors. The same goes for the tiles, which can be geometrically perfect or just slightly off kilter.

We know whose hands these pieces went through: an enthusiastic but unskilled patient, or a gifted woman with time to spend on her work, perhaps because she was going home soon. They also went through the hands of the pottery directors themselves, who used their tenure to practice and perfect their own art.

Arequipa's ceramic history still lives in many private collections (including my own) and at places like the National Museum of American History, the Bancroft Library at the University of California–Berkeley, and the Oakland Museum of California, where Phoebe Brown, Dr. Philip King Brown's daughter, bequeathed her own collection.

Museum visitors can read labels and books to learn the history of Arequipa Pottery, and artists can stand in awe of either the simplicity or complexity of forms and colors as they stare into a display case. But it's difficult today to summon an understanding of how important the pottery was to women who had the chance to take clay into their hands.

Eloise Roorbach, the journalist who visited Arequipa in the spring of 1913, did understand this. Seeing the women at work was a profound personal experience for her. She spent the day talking with the patients and watching them make pottery. She stayed until evening. She reflected about her feelings as she walked to the train station at Manor: "The dark came quickly to the canyon road, but as I stumbled along seeking my way, my thoughts were bright, my heart was warm, for my fingers held tightly a little vase. It was a thing of much importance to me, for it had molded a girl into happiness as surely as her fingers had formed and given it color."[25]

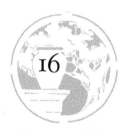

TIME TRAVEL

WHEN MY GRANDMOTHER LOIS DOWNEY went home after her four-teen months at Arequipa, she did her best to put Dr. Cabot Brown's advice—or, to be more accurate, his lecture—into practice.

She was supposed to live quietly and do no household chores for six months. With help from her husband and even her testy mother-in-law, she managed to rest for nearly that long. Little Harvey Jr. had been living with his grandparents nearly the entire time she had been gone, and Lois was worried he might not want to come home. But she underestimated her son, who was now almost four years old. The day she came back from Arequipa, he told his grandmother to move his bed back to his old room with his parents. She protested, she refused, but he would not relent, and he got his way.

Making peace with her mother-in-law was going to be the hardest lesson to follow, but Lois got lucky. A few months after her return to Sonoma, Harvey was transferred to Pacific Gas & Electric Company territory in Sebastopol, about thirty miles to the west. And though she would still see her husband's family at Sunday dinners and other get-togethers, she did not have to do daily battle with Mrs. Downey over how she raised her son.

Lois was not able to stick to one of the cardinal rules for ex-TB patients, however: she got pregnant. This isn't a surprise since she had no access to birth control. (Her son was born just over nine months after she was married.) With hands shaking, she called Cabot Brown, who told her that it was her decision whether or not to go through with the pregnancy. But he told her it would be dangerous for both her and the baby. Even if she did carry the child to term, it would be taken away from her for months to make sure that she was well enough to care for it. The thought of not being able to hold her infant was terrifying. So, heartsick, she decided to get an abortion, which in 1929 was a legal procedure for any woman who had tuberculosis or was recovering from it. Harvey took her on another ferry ride across San Francisco Bay, where she was admitted to St. Francis Hospital, right next door to the medical offices of both Cabot and Philip King Brown. The procedure went well, she went home, and she resettled herself with her family.

She and Harvey were careful this time. She was still under thirty, and once the years progressed, her lungs would heal and pregnancy would no longer be a problem. But when that time came, she was not able to conceive, and she never knew why.

So Lois threw her energies into her only son, and she did the same with her own health. She hadn't taken Arequipa's teachings lightly. She knew that keeping tuberculosis from coming back was entirely up to her and that if she lived the way Dr. Brown told her to, she would stay TB-free. Rather than being oppressive, this concept spurred her into doing only what was good for her, and over the next few decades she went through life like a woman determined to live forever.

~

As the 1950s opened, Lois began to experience symptoms of the arthritis that had nearly crippled her father. She didn't want to end up like he did, and though she took aspirin for the pain, which was in her neck and not her hands, she wanted to try other methods to keep the degeneration at bay. She asked around, read magazines, and decided that massage would be a good idea. Then someone told her about the Seventh-Day Adventist church and college over the hill in the town of Angwin, near Napa. The Adventists believed in traditional medicine and had practitioners she could consult. She called around and found someone who agreed to see her.

Seventh-Day Adventists are vegetarians, and their health practices are an integral part of how they live and minister. They prohibit smoking, drinking, and drugs, and healing is literally hands-on. Lois met the health minister, a Mr. Comer, at his home. He looked her over and recommended a program of massage and vitamins. He also said she should exercise as much as she could, even if she just took a long walk every day. He massaged her neck and she felt so much better afterward that she began to see him regularly.

She also took his advice about food. She wasn't interested in being a vegetarian but thought her family should eat more vegetables anyway. Like many women of her generation, she turned to the canned varieties, grateful that there was a safe and inexpensive alternative to the heavy labor of home canning. She started buying spinach, green beans, and corn at the local market but bought only one brand. From the moment she left Arequipa until the day she left her home for nursing care, the cans on her shelves bore only the S&W label: Sussman & Wormser, the company founded by Blanche Wormser's husband. Blanche died three years before Lois went to Arequipa, but all the patients knew about her and how she had made their lives better. It was a debt Lois needed to repay.

She saw Mr. Comer in Angwin well into the 1960s and followed his advice about food and vitamins the entire time. The massage helped with her arthritis, which fortunately never became debilitating. Whether she knew it consciously or not, the Adventist way of living was as near to the tuberculosis rest cure as you could get outside of a sanatorium. Adventists believe that the body should be given only clean air and water, rest, and good food. More importantly, individuals have to trust in a higher power. My grandmother's instinct for health led her to a method that had helped her before.

The 1950s brought additional joys. In 1950 her son married Evadne Pickering, an Arkansas native who had come out California with her parents during the war so that her father could find work. The two met at San Francisco State College, which Harvey Jr. attended on the GI Bill, thanks to his service in the Pacific during World War II. She became a grandmother with my birth in 1954 and with the birth of my sister, Jan, four years later. The decade was full of parties and camping trips that her sisters- and brothers-in-law enjoyed whenever they had a free weekend, in addition to the occasional bus excursion to the casinos in Reno.

Lois also discovered the fun and exercise benefits of bowling and joined a couple of women's leagues in town. She was soon filling her shelves with tiny trophies. And she particularly enjoyed shopping in a charming new housewares shop run by a lovely young man named Chuck Williams. Everyone in town was tickled when he named his store Williams Sonoma.

~

Lois loved to read, and as America moved closer to the Age of Aquarius in the 1960s, she was intrigued by the many books being published about astrology, meditation, yoga, psychic healing, and other countercultural ideas. In truth, she had always been interested in occult subjects, which explains why she read a book on palmistry when she was at Arequipa. When I was a preteen,

I dove into the same interests and the same books. With every family visit, I raided her shelves to see what new volumes she had added to her pile. We talked about our astrological signs (she Taurus; I Leo) and about how to grow the most important medicinal and ceremonial herbs; Lois also had a gift for gardening. My parents were glad for our close relationship and saw no harm in our mutual interest in subjects they considered a bit wacky, even if the book I enjoyed rereading the most at her house was called *The Black Arts.*

In 1970 Nobel Prize–winning chemist Linus Pauling published *Vitamin C and the Common Cold,* urging Americans to take large doses of the vitamin to prevent colds and to aid their health in general. Mindful of Mr. Comer's many lectures about the value of vitamins, Lois took Pauling's advice and filled her kitchen cabinets with gigantic bottles of vitamin C tablets, which she took regularly. As she was a very active and limber sixty-something, she felt as good as she had twenty years earlier.

In contrast, Harvey's health was deteriorating. He was a smoker and did not subscribe to the food and vitamin regimen that defined Lois's life. In 1972 he developed stomach cancer and died just as I was graduating from high school that June. My grandparents had become distant from each other as they aged and had separate bedrooms by the time I came along. But she still mourned, and then she got on with her life. A couple of years later, a local widower of her acquaintance asked her to go with him on a Caribbean cruise and did not mention separate bedrooms. She declined—not because she wasn't willing to go on a vacation with a man who wasn't her husband but because she just wasn't that fond of him.

I was about five years too young to be a hippie, but I threw myself into the New Age movement of the early 1970s. In 1976 I dropped out of college and joined a small religious cult in San Francisco that was dedicated to meditation, channeling, psychic healing, and vegetarianism. My radical departure shocked everyone in my family except Lois. She wasn't thrilled that I was living in a commune, sleeping on the floor, and selling flowers on the streets of downtown San Francisco, but she didn't try to talk me out of it because she understood the impulse that had made me turn my life over to others. I did something that was very familiar to her: I gave up my free will to an authoritarian figure and lived away from society with a group of people who shared a larger purpose. She did the same thing when she decided to take her health into her hands and live at Arequipa.

A sanatorium has much in common with the way cults are structured to bond people to their beliefs. The first step is to break down the existing self or personality, creating a new identity that is dependent on the leader of the group. Members live in isolated places, and food, sleep, information, and even bodily functions are highly controlled. Leaders use the worship of devotees to build up their egos as much as their institutions. This often leads to rebellion, followed by suppression or expulsion. In a cult, these activities are toxic and abusive. On the surface, they might look the same when they are used at a sanatorium. But unlike cult practices, molding TB patients into new behaviors is for healing and for taking the new self into a new life out in the world.

I escaped from the cult three years later and for a few weeks lived with my parents, who now had a house in Sonoma. I spent most of my time talking with my grandmother. She told me she had gone to a psychic soon after I'd joined the cult and asked him if I was going to be OK. He told her, "Your granddaughter will not do anything that a minister would be ashamed of." (He was wrong, but I didn't tell her that.) A sunny attitude was inherent to her personality, and it had been cultivated into something stronger at Arequipa. Now it was put into service to help me move past my cult years.

Uncovering the Arequipa story and planning for graduate school also helped because I was able to give something back to my grandmother. When I heard that Arequipa was going to be torn down in 1984, I called the *Marin Independent Journal* and told them about her life in the old building. They were intrigued and sent a reporter to Sonoma to interview her. The resulting article included a photo of Lois in full storytelling mode. She clipped it and carried it around for years until it finally crumbled to bits in her purse.

She always looked for ways to shake up her exercise regimen. She started riding a three-wheeled bicycle around Sonoma when she was in her mid-seventies, and she usually carried groceries home in its colorful basket. She also took an aerobics class at the local community center, jumping and twisting to the soundtrack from *Saturday Night Fever*.

When she was eighty, Lois and her friend Betty took a train trip from Oakland to Boston. En route, she fell out of her upper bunk in their sleeping car and was sore for a few days but not permanently damaged. In fact, she never broke a bone in her body until she was in her late eighties; getting out of a rocking chair, she tripped over her Birkenstocks and snapped an ankle. Whether thanks to good genes, exercise, or hormone replacement therapy, she otherwise escaped the fractures common to women of her age, and her ankle healed quickly.

~

My father, sister, and I threw Lois a ninetieth birthday party in 1994. Sturdy and upright, she wolfed down cake and hors d'oeuvres with the large crowd that gathered to celebrate. She still lived alone in senior subsidized housing and still walked every day, though not as much as before. A local woman named Ofelia came in to do the cleaning and help with the cooking. By 1999, however, she needed more help than the few hours Ofelia was able to give her. So she moved in with my father. The inevitable tensions between mother and only son were magnified when they were in the same house, and within a few months Lois came down with pneumonia and had to spend days in a hospital.

She was very sick but managed to pull through, despite her vulnerable lungs. She came out of the hospital clear of infection, but she was no longer able to walk. We then had to make a painful decision. She needed care to get around, to get her meals, and deal with the bathroom. None of this could happen at my father's house, so we admitted her to a highly regarded skilled nursing facility just blocks away from where he lived.

Though woozy from her hospital stay, she knew what was happening. She still had all her marbles and her opinions; it was only her body that was giving out. She didn't seem to understand how much care she really needed and that neither her son nor her granddaughters could manage it. But we visited frequently and tried to keep her spirits up.

A few months after she went into the nursing home, she fell out of bed and broke her hip. She told the doctor she had fallen off her bicycle. She was ninety-five years old, but he decided to do a hip replacement anyway, so she could move around in bed or in her wheelchair without pain. The operation was a success and there were no physical postsurgical complications, but when Lois woke up, she had dropped out of time.

As she slowly recovered from both the anesthesia and the surgery, it was clear she had no idea where she was—in the minds of her doctors and the rest of us, that is. She, however, knew that she was a young wife and mother, little Harvey Jr. was only two, and she had not been felled by tuberculosis. Her room was her Sonoma house, the trees she could see through the window were in her yard, and the tables full of people in the massive dining room at meal times were just friends who had dropped by for lunch or dinner.

The staff had seen this before, but it was a shock for us, as my grandmother had always been lucid. At first this was troubling, because I didn't want to let her go, but one day while I was visiting I had an idea.

I decided to just time travel with her.

Every visit was trip to the past, and though Lois didn't know who I was, she did understand that I was family somehow. I would ask how her day had been, and she would sometimes call out for her toddler son, so I told her he was playing next door. Sometimes when I walked into her room she was having conversations with people I couldn't see, and I figured out that they were long-dead relatives. Once when I came by she said, "Oh, I'm so glad you're here. I want to go fishing, so you can stay here and take care of the cows." I told her I'd be happy to.

She always looked worried when I got ready to leave, so I devised a scheme that would ease her mind. I usually visited after work, when it was dark, so when I needed to go, I asked if I could spend the night, since it was getting late. She would smile and think about which room in the house I could stay in. I then said I was going to my car to get my suitcase, and her smile remained as I passed out of her room. Once I was gone, the memory of my being there also vanished, and so did her concern.

I had to be quick on my feet sometimes. One day I came by about a half hour before dinner. We had a visit and then I wheeled Lois into the dining hall and up to her table, which was occupied by three other women. I told her I had to leave and she asked if I really had to go—couldn't I stay for dinner? I thought for a second and said, "Well, I have a date." She smiled and said, "Oh, of course, you must go." Then, after a moment, she continued, "But try to come back later, because there's going to be dancing."

We brought a cake to the nursing home when she turned one hundred years old in May 2004. When we told her how old she was, she had a moment of clarity and said, "Oh, I can't believe that!" She chuckled as if it were a joke and then went back to demolishing her piece of devil's food cake.

Our father died in 2005, and Jan and I didn't tell her. Lois could not have comprehended the loss of her son, and I had never been more grateful that she found peace in her own past.

Her death just weeks after my husband's passing in 2006 was also incomprehensible to me. As we planned her funeral, I was determined to give the eulogy at the service, which was attended by nieces, nephews, and their own children, spanning multiple generations. And in her honor, I wore red, her favorite color.

My grandmother Lois Bonsey Downey lived the last seventy-seven years of her life as a former TB patient, and they were good years. But when her mind needed to go elsewhere, it chose a time when her lungs were free of disease. She lived to be 102 because Arequipa gave her back her health and taught her how to keep it. But in the end, she preferred the memory of a time when she breathed freely, not knowing what lay ahead.

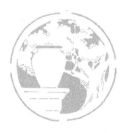

EPILOGUE

IN SEPTEMBER 2015 I went back to Arequipa for the first time in nearly thirty years. I wanted to write a book about my grandmother's experience and thought that retracing the steps I'd taken with her so long before would be inspiring.

I wasn't sure I could even get onto the property, though. Girl Scout events were winding down, but I knew that other groups rented the land to hold conferences and seminars. It was worth a try, so I left my Sonoma County home and headed south to Marin.

I took the two-lane road west from Fairfax and a few miles later saw the stone entryway that Henry Bothin had donated to the sanatorium a century earlier. Luck was with me; the iron gates were wide open. I drove in and noticed a large tent set up near the main parking lot. I could hear voices coming from inside, so I maneuvered slowly past it and up the hill to where the old buildings used to be, as if I owned the place.

I parked my car and spied the Philip King Brown memorial bench in a patch of deep shade. The granite was mossy and slightly pitted, but the tile marker was bright. Steps next to the bench led up a hill to a small overhang marked as a campsite.

I walked farther up the driveway and saw that the sanatorium's concrete foundations were still there, left behind after the building's demolition in 1984. Below these was a cleared area with more old cement underpinnings, and I headed toward them down a steeply inclined path. I then heard a noise behind me and turned to see a gigantic black-tailed deer, a two-point buck, standing at the top of the walkway, letting me know with one look that I was in his territory. I turned to leave, aiming for a trail that went in the opposite direction, but my movement made him swivel and bound away.

Alone again, I discovered that the tile-covered concrete bench that used to encircle a corner of the old tiled patio was still there—chipped, darkened, and covered with leaves, but firmly in place. The hydrangea bush from my grandmother's 1929 photo was gone, and so was the patio itself.

As I sat on one of the concrete pilings and took in the same scents that had filled me on my first childhood visit, I recalled how Arequipa always seemed to resurface in my life. Serendipity often follows writers who are committed to a book, or even the idea of one, and it started trailing me the day I returned to Arequipa as an adult. It's the reason you are holding this volume in your hands.

~

When I began my research back in 1983, I thought that some of Arequipa's former patients might still be alive, so I placed ads in the Marin County paper, the *Independent Journal*. That's how I found Patty and Bonnie, who were both happy to give me their stories. In 1984 I also found Phoebe Hearst Brown, Philip and Helen's only daughter, who still lived in the family home her parents built after the earthquake and fire.

I wrote her a letter introducing myself and said that I would like to ask some questions about her father and the sanatorium. She wrote back, agreeing to a meeting and inviting me to her house. She was a formidable woman: stout and gray-haired, she had the strong features of her grandmother Charlotte, with the character to match. She told me she was blind (her letter had been dictated to a secretary), so I was expecting that, but if I expected a woman who thought she was disabled, I was soon proved wrong.

She moved around her home without difficulty, but if she did need help, a man named James Tong Lee was close by. He had worked for the family since the late 1930s or so and was always known as Mr. Lee. He got the both of us settled after my arrival: Phoebe in a window seat that overlooked the Golden Gate and me in a nearby chair. She then proceeded to interview me before I could even get started with my questions, and I quaked as I explained further why I wanted to talk with her.

As I told her about my grandmother and how Arequipa had saved her life, Brown began to thaw, and we had an enjoyable and productive time together. I knew she had trained as an architect and had a career as a planner with the city of San Francisco, and I asked her why she chose that profession. She replied, "Because I would look at buildings and think to myself, 'I could do better than that.'"

We exchanged letters well into 1989, and she always answered my questions or pointed me toward a new area of research. I was grateful that I'd found her and for all she gave me. She died in November 1990.

One important area of my research was the pottery, which had its own experts in the ceramics world. Chief among them were Joe Taylor and Sheila Menzies, who run the Tile Heritage Foundation, a nonprofit dedicated to saving and sharing information about historic ceramic tile. They found me in 1987 thanks to one of my early articles and gave me piles of material to work with as I studied Dr. Brown's experiment in occupational therapy.

In the mid-1980s I worked for a few months at a temporary job agency in Marin County, interviewing prospective employees for the firm's clients. One day a tall, thin older man came in and sat down at my desk. He filled out an application, and when I saw that his last name was Solon, I quipped, "You aren't any relation to Albert Solon are you?" As I laughed at my silly joke and began to make some notes on his paperwork, he said, "Yes, I am."

I stared at him as he smiled. I'm sure I looked like a complete idiot for a moment. Then I pulled myself together and explained why I had asked the question: I was researching the Arequipa Pottery, Albert Solon was the second director, and so on. He turned out to be one of Albert's nephews. We traded phone numbers, and he invited me to his home in San Francisco. I visited a couple of weeks later, and over coffee and cookies he gave me personal details about his uncle that I would never have found elsewhere. My favorite story was about Albert's efforts to grow hair when he started balding later in life. He bought a black cap with an ultraviolet light inside that was supposed to stimulate hair growth as he wore it.

One day about this same time, while I was looking up information about Bruce Porter, Dr. Brown's friend and artistic adviser, I read about his designs for Joseph Worcester's Swedenborgian Church in San Francisco. The name rang a bell, and then it hit me: my parents were married in Worcester's church in July 1950 as the sun streamed through Porter's stained-glass windows.

I put Arequipa aside in the late 1990s as I concentrated on my career and other research projects. But it always found its way back to me. In 2000, just as my husband was diagnosed with the cancer that would take his life, the Oakland Museum opened a major exhibition of Arequipa pottery and I was invited to write the historical essay for the catalog. It was a distraction I desperately needed. Then, with the loss of my grandmother and my retirement from corporate life, I knew it was time to make her story a priority again.

~

One January day in 2018, I checked my email and saw that someone named Sarah Brown had written to me via my website. Sarah, who lives in Washington, D.C., turned out to be Philip King Brown's great-granddaughter and the granddaughter of Cabot Brown, my grandmother's doctor during her time at Arequipa. Sarah found me while wandering around the internet, looking for information about the sanatorium. We began to correspond like old friends and sent historical information back and forth. I also traded emails with her sister, Charlotte, who lived on the East Coast too. I loved writing to someone named Charlotte Brown after spending so much time writing *about* someone named Charlotte Brown.

Later that spring, Sarah emailed to tell me that her brother, Andrew, and his fiancée, Olga, would be visiting California in May from their home in New York. They were planning to see friends in a town about an hour from my home and hoped that I was free for lunch. Well, of course I was. So on a beautiful sunny Saturday I walked into the restaurant and told the hostess I was with the Andrew Brown party. She motioned me to the back of a crowded patio. I'd never met Andrew, but when I walked toward a group of tables, I knew him immediately: he had the same features I'd been seeing in historical photos for three decades.

As we enjoyed our long lunch, Andrew and Olga were content to let me babble on about how I got interested in Arequipa, but we also had something else to talk about. Two months earlier, I'd found another former patient.

In early March I had received an email from a Dr. Michael Thompson. He told me about an elderly woman named Rose whom he treated when he was on the faculty of George Washington University Medical School in Washington, D.C. The two of them kept in touch, even when he relocated to the University of Massachusetts Medical School in Worcester. Whenever they chatted, she told him about the years she spent at a California tuberculosis sanatorium called Arequipa. Dr. Thompson wanted to know more about the place, and, like Sarah, he found me online. He said that Rose wanted to talk to me about her experience. I replied that I would be thrilled. He gave me her phone number, and I called her the very next day.

During our short introductory phone call, I quickly realized that this ninety-one-year-old woman not only had perfectly sharp memories of her time at Arequipa, but her mind was sharp about everything else. A few days later we had a two-hour conversation as she spun out her stories and I took pages of notes. It didn't take long for us to become weekly phone-call buddies. Funny, politically savvy, and engaged, Rose always made me laugh out loud at least once during our chats. I introduced Rose and Sarah to each other, as it turned out, they lived just three miles apart in Washington. Rose also put me in touch with her niece Carole, who lived in San Francisco. As the weeks went by and I got to know Rose better, I began to feel that some part of my grandmother had come back to me.

∾

When I made my pilgrimage to Arequipa in the fall of 2015, I expected it to be my last. By early 2018 I was putting the finishing touches on this book and believed that with its completion, the sanatorium as physical place would give way to the sanatorium as printed book, the one I always wanted to write. After finding Rose and the Brown family, I thought that the empty site would no longer play a role in my life. Arequipa had given me everything it possibly could. But I was wrong.

A few weeks after I started talking with Rose, Sarah emailed to say that she was coming out to California in mid-June to visit her Bay Area relatives. She had never been to Arequipa and wondered if I could take her to see the property. Her cousin Margot also wanted to go; she was the daughter of Bruce Brown, Helen and Philip's youngest child. She lived in one of the East Bay cities outside San Francisco and had gone to Arequipa in 1980 when she dropped off her daughter Alyson for a Girl Scout outing. Margot had been astonished to see the Philip King Brown memorial bench there, because she had no idea her grandfather had built the very place she was standing in. Neither she nor Alyson had been back since, and Alyson also wanted to come along.

Since it was summer, I knew the Girl Scouts would probably be running their camp activities. And I didn't think we could just wander in (trespass) like I'd done before. So I jumped onto the Girl Scout website and confirmed that a day camp would be in full swing when Sarah and her cousins wanted to visit. I emailed the local Girl Scout organization and said that I would like to bring some of Dr. Philip King Brown's descendants on a visit to Arequipa, and would that be OK? I got a reply right away from a woman named Sharon Sagar, who happened to be president of the Fairfax Historical Society and was familiar with my research.

She sent my request up the chain to the leaders in charge of the June camp, and they immediately said yes. I also offered to give the Scouts a short talk about

Arequipa's history. This made our visit even more enticing, and they invited us to stay for lunch.

I met Sarah, Margot, and Alyson at the Good Earth natural foods store in Fairfax on a clear, cool June morning and then drove us out to Arequipa. Brian Sagar, Sharon's husband and the former president of the Fairfax Historical Society, met us at the parking lot. The day camp's organizers also greeted us and said to wander at our leisure but to be sure to come down to the campfire ring in time for lunch. We set off, with Brian in the lead. His deep knowledge of Arequipa's history complemented mine, and we gave the three women a full historical tour. We both took photos of two generations of Browns sitting on the memorial bench.

The leaders then gathered up the Scouts, about seventy-five of them, all in matching T-shirts and ranging in age from grade school to high school. I stood in front of the group, and as they ate their lunch, I gave a quick talk about Dr. Brown and his sanatorium, passing around copies of some historical pictures. The girls not only paid close attention; they also asked very thoughtful questions when I was finished, including a sweet one from a girl who wanted to know if my grandmother was still alive. Then it was time for the adults to eat, and we enjoyed our Caesar salad, rolls, and Girl Scout cookies while we chatted with some of the local troop's earliest leaders, who had been specially invited for the occasion.

Before this visit I had started to formulate a plan with Andrew and Sarah. They knew I wanted to meet Rose and hear her story in person. But they also knew that a trip to Washington, D.C., was beyond my budget. No problem: Andrew and Olga would pay for my airline ticket, and Sarah would put me up. The deal was done before I could say no.

I spent six days in D.C. and stayed with Sarah and her husband, Alan, who gave me the pick of the guest rooms in their beautiful home near the National Cathedral. I spent three of those days with Rose in her apartment complex near the Watergate. She was as sprightly in person as she was on the phone. She was dressed in soft gray slacks and a black top with two large pink flowers on the front, which perfectly matched her lipstick. Her smile was wider than mine, and we had a quick chat before going upstairs to a friend's vacant apartment.

Her niece Maura was visiting from Michigan and was staying in the apartment while Rose's friends were out of town. She had brought a video camera so she could record my interview with her Auntie Rose and share it with the family. We sat at the dining table and talked for nearly an hour and a half, and she added some juicy details to the stories she had told me during our telephone chats. As we ended the interview, Rose mused about what Arequipa had done for her, what it had meant to her: "Everyone was very loving. They gave me a home, health care, and friendship, without demanding any return."

Even when I wasn't with Rose during the Washington trip, Arequipa was still with me. I took one day just for the museums on the Mall and made a beeline for the National Museum of American History, where I'd seen examples of Arequipa pottery on my last visit about twelve years earlier. But I got a shock when I walked through the door: the museum had been thoroughly renovated, and although I found a nice collection of art pottery in the *Art & Industry* exhibit, there was no Arequipa pottery on the shelves.

I cheered up when I saw a temporary exhibit called *Modern Medicine and the Great War*. The small display included a nurse's uniform, probably the same type Emma Applegren had worn in France during her stint there during World War I. The curators had also put in examples of beadwork and pottery made by wounded soldiers as rehabilitation therapy. These reminded me of the three young women from the University of California who had come to Arequipa in the spring of 1918 as "reconstruction aides," perfecting their skills by teaching beadwork and weaving to the patients.

But that wasn't all. I wandered into the military history section of the museum and found a docent standing behind a table covered with World War I objects for visitors to actually handle. Among these were a cup made especially for men with facial wounds and what looked like an oversize cribbage board whose removable pegs helped men regain their hand coordination. I held both of these for a long time, thinking about Arequipa's small contribution to relieving suffering outside its own walls.

I also went to the National Museum of the American Indian. Among the exhibits was a look at the Quechua culture of Peru, which intrigued me because the name *Arequipa* came from that part of the world. As I read the interesting explanatory panels, I came across a section that stopped me in my tracks.

In the Quechua language there are no words to express the future; there are only terms for past and present. I stood in front of the exhibit blocking traffic as this information took hold in my mind. It perfectly expressed life at Arequipa Sanatorium, where the future was so hazy that it barely existed. There was only the past, when TB came into a woman's life and lungs, and only the present, while she battled to vanquish it. Philip King Brown had picked the perfect name for his life's work.

~

I went back to Arequipa twice when I was in my early sixties, with decades of life experience and books about other topics behind me. On both of these visits I went through the gates expecting to feel melancholy when I left.

But I didn't.

Somehow it was still *my* Arequipa. It belonged to me even before my ten-year-old self first saw it and felt the mesmerizing power of the old building. It was part of my family decades before I was born. It lived in my continued friendship with Happy and Cari Lyn Stanton. And it thrived in the circle of new friends it brought me: Sarah and Alan, Andrew and Olga, Charlotte, Margot, Alyson, and, of course, Rose and her extended family.

I also knew that the Girl Scouts told troops about Arequipa's history, and perhaps a few girls thought about the sanatorium as they sat on Dr. Brown's bench. As a historian, I know that institutions live on even when buildings have gone to rot and all memory has fled. They live through the people who served or were healed there, and they can even exert intangible, lingering benefits. Arequipa was no exception. Its influence extended into the lives of the women who walked its wards and its grounds—and even those who didn't.

Life at Arequipa was about waiting for breath to return as lungs were healed, and for nearly fifty years the sanatorium asked just one thing of its patients. It was a simple prescription, a calm admonition from doctors who fought TB every day of their working lives.

Here, rest.

GLOSSARY

bacillus: a type of bacterium that causes diseases such as tuberculosis. The plural is *bacilli*.

bronchoscopy: a procedure in which a scope goes into the trachea to look at the bronchi of the lungs. The bronchi are airway passages of the pulmonary system.

empyema: a bacterial infection in the pleural cavity around the lung.

fluoroscope: a medical imaging system that uses X-ray technology to capture the inner workings of the body. In sanatoria, fluoroscopes were used to look at lung function as patients were being treated, to monitor their progress.

macrophages: the scar tissue that forms around clusters of tubercular bacilli in the lungs as a patient takes the rest cure. These remain in the lungs even after the person is no longer contagious.

pneumolysis: a procedure in which adhesions in the pleural cavity surrounding a lung are surgically removed, to allow the lung to collapse and to facilitate healing.

pneumothorax: the most common treatment in tuberculosis sanatoria. Nitrogen is injected into the pleural cavity to artificially collapse a lung, which allows it to rest and allows macrophages to form around the bacilli.

thoracoplasty: a procedure used in more serious cases of tuberculosis. One or more ribs are removed so that a lung will permanently collapse, which can speed healing because the lung is not being used.

up: ambulatory. In sanatoria, up patients were allowed to get out of bed and move around because they were no longer contagious. Their up time was a way to gauge their readiness to go home.

NOTES

CHAPTER 1. THE MAVERICK

1. Helen Hillyer Brown, *The Great San Francisco Fire* (San Francisco: Leo Holub, 1956), passim.
2. Adelaide Brown, "The History of the Development of Women in Medicine in California." *California and Western Medicine* 23 (May 1925): 579–80.
3. Charles Morris Blake to Rev. A. S. Packard, D.D., March 22, 1879, Sharlot Hall Museum, Prescott, Arizona.
4. *Arizona Weekly Journal-Miner*, October 13, 1866.
5. *Arizona Weekly Journal-Miner*, January 12, 1867.
6. *Arizona Weekly Journal-Miner*, May 9, 1866.
7. *Arizona Weekly Journal-Miner*, August 10, 1867.
8. Adelaide Brown, "The History of the Development of Women in Medicine in California," 580.
9. Howard Markel, "Celebrating Rebecca Lee Crumpler, First African-American Woman Physician," *PBS New Hour*, March 9, 2016, https://www.pbs.org /newshour/health/celebrating-rebecca-lee-crumpler-first-african-american -physician (accessed December 7, 2018).
10. Regina Markell Morantz-Sanchez, *Sympathy and Science: Women Physicians in American Medicine* (New York: Oxford, 1985), 29–31, 48–50, 52–53.
11. Henry Harris, *California's Medical Story* (San Francisco: Grabhorn Press, 1932), 132–36.
12. Morantz-Sanchez, *Sympathy and Science*, 101.
13. Adelaide Brown, "The History of the Development of Women in Medicine in California," 580.
14. Morantz-Sanchez, *Sympathy and Science,* 48–49, 68.
15. Harris, *California's Medical Story,* 208.
16. Adelaide Brown, "The History of the Development of Women in Medicine in California," 579.
17. *San Francisco Chronicle,* June 23, 1873.

CHAPTER 2. THE DRS. BROWN

1. Mark Twain, *Roughing It* (Hartford, Conn.: American Publishing Company, 1982), 420.
2. *Report of the Health Officer of the City and County of San Francisco for the Fiscal Year Ending June 30, 1875* (San Francisco: Spaulding and Barto, 1875), 7.

3. San Francisco city directories and corporate records, Wells, Fargo & Co. Archives, San Francisco.

4. H. E. Thelander, "Children's Hospital of San Francisco," *Medical Woman's Journal* (July 1934): 184–98.

5. James K. Brown, "Growing Up: 1937–1939" (unpublished memoir).

6. Meredith Eliassen, "The San Francisco Experiment: Female Medical Practitioners Caring for Women and Children, 1875–1935," *Gender Forum* 25 (2009): 2.

7. *San Francisco Call*, May 7, 1894.

8. Judith Robinson, *The Hearsts: An American* Dynasty (New York: Avon, 1991), 31–56, 162–65, 238.

9. Oscar Lewis, *Bay Window Bohemia: An Account of the Brilliant Artistic World of Gaslit San Francisco* (Garden City, N.Y.: Doubleday, 1956), 81–82.

10. *San Francisco Call*, January 3, 1894.

11. Birgitta Hjalmarson, *Artful Players: Artistic Life in Early San Francisco* (Los Angeles: Balcony Press, 1999): 179.

12. *New York Times*, May 15, 1895.

13. Lawrence Dinnean, *Les Jeunes: An Account of Some Fin de Siècle San Francisco Authors and Artists* (Berkeley: Friends of the Bancroft Library, 1980), 1–5.

14. Frank Norris Collection of Papers and Related Materials, Bancroft Library, University of California–Berkeley.

15. San Francisco Polyclinic, *Annual Report* (San Francisco: San Francisco Polyclinic, 1892), 3.

16. Philip King Brown to Phoebe Apperson Hearst, April 5, 1899, Bancroft Library, University of California–Berkeley.

17. Helen Hillyer Brown, *For My Children and Grandchildren* (San Francisco: Hillside Press, 1986).

18. Philip King Brown to Phoebe Apperson Hearst, March 27, 1900, Bancroft Library, University of California–Berkeley.

19. Brown to Hearst, March 27, 1900.

20. *San Francisco Call*, February 6, February 10, February 27, March 5, May 8, June 29, 1904; *San Francisco Chronicle,* May 25, 1905.

CHAPTER 3. CONSUMED

1. Helen Hillyer Brown, *Great San Francisco Fire*, passim.

2. *Los Angeles Herald*, January 10, 1908.

3. Mary Hotaling, *A Rare Romance in Medicine: The Life and Legacy of Edward Livingston Trudeau* (Saranac Lake, N.Y.: Historic Saranac Lake, 2016), 80–81.

4. Hotaling, *A Rare Romance in Medicine*, 3–95, passim.

5. *San Francisco Call*, August 19, 1908.

6. Philip King Brown, "Outdoor Life in California," *Journal of the Outdoor Life* 15 (March 1908): 45–48.

7. Philip King Brown, "Tuberculosis Class Work in the San Francisco Polyclinic," *Merchants' Association Review* 14 (September 1909): 5–6.

8. Heather Cox Richardson, *West from Appomattox: The Reconstruction of America after the Civil War* (New Haven, Conn.: Yale University Press, 2007), 80–81.

9. Barbara Mayer Wertheimer, *We Were There: The Story of Working Women in America* (New York: Pantheon Books, 1977), 156–68.

10. National Tuberculosis Association, *Transactions of the Fourteenth Annual Meeting, June 6–8, 1918* (New York: National Tuberculosis Association, 1919), 436.

11. Jules Tygiel, *Workingmen in San Francisco, 1880–1901* (New York: Garland, 1992), 23.

12. Wertheimer, *We Were There*, 237.

13. *San Francisco Call*, October 1, 1905.

14. Brown, "Tuberculosis Class Work," 6.

15. Paul Groth, *Living Downtown: The History of Residential Hotels in the United States* (Berkeley: University of California Press, 1994), 90–130, passim.

16. *San Francisco Call*, January 22, 1905.

17. Groth, *Living Downtown*, 205–6.

CHAPTER 4. PROGRESSIVES

1. Charlotte Brown, "The Health of Our Girls," paper presented to the Medical Society of the State of California, Los Angeles, April 1896.

2. *San Francisco Call*, March 22, 1901.

3. National Association for the Study and Prevention of Tuberculosis, *A Tuberculosis Directory: A List of Institutions, Associations and Other Agencies Dealing with Tuberculosis in the United States and Canada* (New York: National Association for the Study and Prevention of Tuberculosis, 1911), 13, 15.

4. Michael Casey, *Henry E. Bothin: Philanthropist of Steel* (Nicasio, Calif.: Michael Casey, 2015), 89–225.

5. Henry Bothin to Elizabeth Ashe, December 27, 1910 (letter owned by Andrew Brown).

6. Richard Hofstadter, *The Progressive Movement, 1900–1915* (Englewood Cliffs, N.J.: Prentice-Hall, 1963), 2.

7. Kathryn Kish Sklar, "The 'Quickened Conscience': Women's Voluntarism and the State, 1890–1920," *Institute for Philosophy and Public Policy Quarterly* 18 (1998): 27–33.

8. Edward Livingston Trudeau, "The Part of Women in Tuberculosis Work," *Journal of the Outdoor Life* 6 (April 1909): 92.

CHAPTER 5. HERE, REST

1. Peter Hartmann and Stacey Wright, "Muy Rico Channel Drive," *Santa Barbara Urban Hikers*, April 21, 2012, http://santabarbaraurbanhikers.com/151/muy-rico-channel-drive (accessed December 7, 2018).

2. *Los Angeles Times*, December 22, 1912; *Los Angeles Times*, October 31, 1915.

3. Arequipa Sanatorium, *Annual Report* (Fairfax, Calif.: Arequipa Sanatorium, 1912), 12.

4. *San Francisco Call*, November 11, 1910.

5. Arequipa Sanatorium, *Annual Report*, 1912, 12.

6. Jewish Museum of the American West, "Isaac Wormser Family, San Francisco Jewish Pioneers & Founder of S&W Fine Foods," *Jewish Museum of the American West*, March 1, 2013, http://www.jmaw.org/wormser-jewish-san-francisco/ (accessed December 7, 2018).

7. *Argonaut*, July 6, 1912.

8. *Marin Journal*, May 4, 1905.

9. Isabel Dibblee to Philip King Brown, undated, Bancroft Library, University of California–Berkeley.

10. *San Francisco Call*, November 21, 1910.

11. Philip King Brown to Phoebe Apperson Hearst, October 17, 1910, Bancroft Library, University of California–Berkeley.

12. Philip King Brown to Phoebe Apperson Hearst, July 27, 1911, Bancroft Library, University of California–Berkeley.

13. Arequipa Sanatorium, *Annual Report*, 1912, 2.

14. *San Francisco Chronicle*, May 20, 1912; *San Francisco Chronicle*, June 20, 1912.

15. Douglas Henry Daniels, *Pioneer Urbanites: A Social and Cultural History of Black San Francisco* (Philadelphia: Temple University Press, 1980), 23.

16. Albert S. Broussard, *Black San Francisco: The Struggle for Racial Equality in the West, 1900–1954* (Lawrence: University Press of Kansas, 1993), 59.

17. Thomas Spees Carrington, *Tuberculosis Hospital and Sanatorium Construction* (New York: National Association for the Study and Prevention and Tuberculosis, 1914), 17.

18. W. Jarvis Barlow to Philip King Brown, November 4, 1910, Bancroft Library, University of California–Berkeley.

19. Richard Longstreth, *On the Edge of the World: Four Architects in San Francisco at the Turn of the Century* (New York: Architectural History Foundation, 1983), 297.

20. *San Francisco Call*, January 12, 1912.

21. W. Jarvis Barlow to Philip King Brown, November 4, 1910, Bancroft Library, University of California–Berkeley.

22. *San Francisco Chronicle*, April 6, 1911.

23. Edward Livingston Trudeau to Philip King Brown, October 26, 1911.

24. Stephen Fried, *Appetite for America: How Visionary Businessman Fred Harvey Built a Railroad Hospitality Empire That Civilized the Wild West* (New York: Random House, 2010), 259.

25. Pryce Mitchell, *Deep Water: The Autobiography of a Sea Captain* (Boston: Little, Brown, 1933), 312.

26. Arequipa Sanatorium, *Annual Report*, 1912, 7.

CHAPTER 6. ART AS A TONIC

1. Broussard, *Black San Francisco*, 53–54.

2. *Denver Medical Times* 18, no. 2 (August 1898): 26; *Los Angeles Times*, August 3, 1904; *Denver Post*, April 28, 1906; United States Census, 1910.

3. Arequipa Sanatorium, *Annual Report* (Fairfax, Calif.: Arequipa Sanatorium, 1913), 7.

4. United States Census, 1920.

5. *Alumni Directory and Ten-Year Book, 1891–1910* (Stanford, Calif.: Stanford University, 1910), 175.

6. Poetry file, Arequipa Collection, Bancroft Library, University of California–Berkeley.

7. Paul Evans, *Art Pottery of the United States* (New York: Feingold and Lewis, 1987), 157–60.

8. Richard Guy Wilson, "'Divine Excellence': The Arts and Crafts Life in California," in *The Arts and Crafts Movement in California: Living the Good Life*, ed. Kenneth Trapp (New York: Abbeville Press, 1993), 17.

9. Evans, *Art Pottery of the United States*, 54–55, 182–87, 213–16, 243–49, 255–57.

10. Helen Hillyer Brown, "The History of the Arequipa Pottery," 1914, Arequipa Collection, Bancroft Library, University of California–Berkeley.

11. Sharon Dale, *Frederick Hurten Rhead: An English Potter in America* (Erie, Pa.: Erie Art Museum, 1986), 10–90, passim.

12. Durlynn Anema, *Ynes Mexia: Botanist and Adventurer* (Greensboro, N.C.: Morgan Reynolds Publishing, 2005), 13–24.

13. Leslie M. Freudenheim, "Icon of Simplicity: The American Arts & Crafts Movement Started at the Swedenborgian Church," *Center for Swedenborgian Studies of the Graduate Theological Union*, https://css.gtu.edu/icon-of-simplicity/ (accessed December 7, 2018).

14. Author interview with Phoebe Hearst Brown, 1984.

15. *San Francisco Call*, August 17, 1913.

16. Author interview with Phoebe Hearst Brown, 1984.

17. *San Francisco Call*, October 27, 1912.

18. Eloise Roorbach, "Art as a Tonic," *Craftsman* 24 (June 1913): 343–46.

19. United States Census, 1880, 1900; Alameda County directories, 1908, 1912; Arequipa Sanatorium, *Annual Report*, 1912, 16.

20. Philip King Brown to Ynés Mexía, July 23, 1912, Bancroft Library, University of California–Berkeley.

21. Nora Harnden to Philip King Brown, undated, Bancroft Library, University of California–Berkeley.

22. *San Francisco Call*, January 22, 1913.

23. Nora Harnden to Philip King Brown, July 10, 1913, Bancroft Library, University of California–Berkeley.

CHAPTER 7. TILE AND TROUBLE

1. Arequipa pottery pamphlet, Arequipa Collection, Bancroft Library, University of California–Berkeley.

2. Evans, *Art Pottery of the United States*, 17–18.

3. Helen Hillyer Brown, "The History of the Arequipa Pottery."

4. *Marin Journal*, April 23, 1914.

5. United States Census, 1900; Arequipa Sanatorium, *Annual Report* (Fairfax, Calif.: Arequipa Sanatorium, 1915), 24.

6. Joseph A. Taylor, "Creating Beauty from the Earth: The Tiles of California," in Trapp, *The Arts and Crafts Movement in California*, 111–15.

7. Arequipa Sanatorium, *Annual Report* (Fairfax, Calif.: Arequipa Sanatorium, 1917), 19–20.

8. *Philadelphia Enquirer*, February 12, 1911; Amilu S. Rothhammer, "A Lofty Mountain to Scale: A Tale of Perseverance," *Archives of Surgery Journal* 136 (May 2001): 501; *Woman's Medical Journal* 16 (October 1906): 163.

9. Nora Harnden to Philip King Brown, undated, Bancroft Library, University of California–Berkeley.

10. Nora Harnden to Philip King Brown, undated; probably August 1917, Bancroft Library, University of California–Berkeley.

11. Poetry in Arequipa Collection, Bancroft Library, University of California–Berkeley.

12. Nora Harnden to Philip King Brown, November 3, 1917, Bancroft Library, University of California–Berkeley.

13. Ynés Mexia Papers, Bancroft Library, University of California–Berkeley.

14. Richard C. Cabot, "Arequipa Sanatorium: Where a Tuberculous Patient Can Be Cured without Expense to Himself or Anyone Else," *Survey*, December 7, 1912; *San Francisco Call*, January 24, 1909; *San Francisco Call*, February 1, 1909.

15. *Oakland Tribune*, November 12, 1916.

16. Robinson, *The Hearsts*, 307–8, 363.

17. *San Francisco Chronicle*, September 11, 1911; *San Francisco Chronicle*, December 14, 1915.

18. *Directory of Physicians and Surgeons, Osteopaths, Drugless Practitioners, Chiropodists, Midwives* (Sacramento: Board of Medical Examiners of the State of California, 1918); Arequipa Sanatorium, *Annual Report* (Fairfax, Calif.: Arequipa Sanatorium, 1919), 11.

19. Philip King Brown, "Interesting Comments from Paris," *California State Journal of Medicine* 17 (January 1919): 29.

20. Philip King Brown to Ynés Mexía, October 18, 1918, Bancroft Library, University of California–Berkeley.

21. *San Anselmo Herald*, June 30, 1921.

22. *San Anselmo Herald*, September 10, 1915.

CHAPTER 8. LIFE IN A LUNG RESORT

1. Arequipa Sanatorium, *Annual Report* (Fairfax, Calif.: Arequipa Sanatorium, 1922), 25.

2. United States Census, 1910; San Francisco city directory, 1912.

3. Jennifer A. Bloom Hoover, "Diversional Occupational Therapy in World War I: A Need for Purpose in Occupations," *American Journal of Occupational Therapy* 50 (November/December 1996): 882.

4. Arequipa Sanatorium, *Annual Report* 1919, 17–19.

5. Arequipa Sanatorium, *Annual Report*, 1922, 28.

6. Society of Arts and Crafts of Boston, *Annual Report* (Boston: Society of Arts and Crafts, 1918); "New and Noteworthy Collections," Special Collections, University of California–Irvine; *Variety*, October 14, 1942, 3; *Los Angeles Times*, January 31, 1940.

7. "The Need of a Post-Graduate School for Nurses," *Proceedings, Seventeenth Annual Conference of Charities and Corrections, 1890* (Boston: Geo. H. Ellis, 1890), 152.

8. Patricia D'Antonio, *American Nursing: A History of Knowledge, Authority, and the Meaning of Work* (Baltimore: Johns Hopkins University Press, 2010), 12–45, passim.

9. Theodore B. Sachs, "The Tuberculosis Nurse," *American Journal of Nursing* (May 1908): 597.

10. United States Census, 1900; Hospital for Children and Training School for Nurses, *Annual Report* (San Francisco: Hospital for Children and Training School for Nurses, 1906), 77.

11. Sister Rose Genevieve, "Diet in Tuberculosis," *Journal of the Outdoor Life* 25 (January 1928): 15.

12. Harry Lee Barnes, "Food Complaints in Sanatoria," *Journal of the Outdoor Life* 25 (January 1928): 13–14.

13. Arequipa Sanatorium, *Annual Report*, 1919, 16.

14. Arequipa Sanatorium, *Annual Report*, 1919, 16–17.

15. Poetry in Arequipa Collection, Bancroft Library, University of California–Berkeley.

16. Susan Craddock, *City of Plagues: Disease, Poverty, and Deviance in San Francisco* (Minneapolis: University of Minnesota Press, 2000), 178.

17. "Rules and Information for Patients," Arequipa Collection, Bancroft Library, University of California–Berkeley.

18. Craddock, *City of Plagues*, 179.

19. Craddock, *City of Plagues*, 179.

20. Arequipa Sanatorium, *Annual Report*, 1919, 14–15.

CHAPTER 9. TO HER THE GIRLS COULD BRING THEIR TROUBLES

1. Nili Tannenbaum and Michael Reisch, "From Charitable Volunteers to Architects of Social Welfare: A Brief History of Social Work," *Ongoing* (Fall 2001): 6–11.

2. Arequipa Sanatorium, *Annual Report*, 1915, 15.

3. Arequipa Sanatorium, *Annual Report* (Fairfax, Calif.: Arequipa Sanatorium, 1916), 11.

4. United States Census, 1880; *Daily Alta California*, May 26, 1885; *Oakland Tribune*, May 17, 1899; San Francisco city directories, 1900–1913; Arequipa Sanatorium, *Annual Report*, 1915, 14–15.

5. United States Census, 1880; Arequipa Sanatorium, *Annual Report*, 1917, 15–16.

6. Arequipa Sanatorium, *Annual Report*, 1919, 22; Arequipa Sanatorium, *Annual Report*, 1922, 16.

7. Arequipa Sanatorium, *Annual Report*, 1922, 18.

8. Arequipa Sanatorium, *Annual Report* (Fairfax, Calif.: Arequipa Sanatorium, 1924), 7.

9. United States Census, 1910; *Stanford Daily*, November 17, 1944; U.S. Department of Labor, Immigration Service, "List of United States Citizens (for the Immigration Authorities)," November 20, 1924, *Ancestry.com*, https://search.ancestry.com/cgi-bin /sse.dll?indiv=1&dbid=7488&h=4028738727&tid=&pid=&usePUB=true&_phsrc =bbT1486&_phstart=successSource (accessed January 9, 2019).

10. *San Francisco Chronicle*, September 26, 1921.

11. U.S. Department of Commerce and Labor, Immigration Service, "List or Manifest of Alien Passengers for the United States," July 19, 1913, *Ancestry.com*, https://search.ancestry.com/cgi-bin/sse.dll?indiv=1&dbid=7949&h=278900&tid=&pid=&usePUB=true&_phsrc=bbT1503&_phstart=successSource (accessed January 9, 2019); U.S. Department of Labor, Immigration Service, "List or Manifest of Alien Passengers for the United States," December 7, 1919, *Ancestry*.com, https://search.ancestry.com/cgi-bin/sse.dll?indiv=1&dbid=7949&h=102949&tid=&pid=&usePUB=true&_phsrc=bbT1506&_phstart=successSource (accessed January 9, 2019); United States Census, 1920; California State Library, "Great Register of Voters," 1900–1968, *Ancestry.com*, https://search.ancestry.com/cgi-bin/sse.dll?_phsrc=bbT1514&_phstart=successSource&usePUBJs=true&indiv=1&db=cavoterrosetta&gsfn=elizabeth&gsln=macmillan&msrpn__ftp=marin,%20california,%20usa&msrpn=1886&new=1&rank=1&redir=false&uidh=d56&gss=angs-d&pcat=35&fh=12&h=60324410&recoff=&ml_rpos=13 (accessed January 9, 2019); author interview with Rose.

12. *Hi-Life*, September 12, 1921, Arequipa Collection, Bancroft Library, University of California–Berkeley.

13. *Hi-Life*, September 12, 1922, Arequipa Collection, Bancroft Library, University of California–Berkeley.

14. *Hi-Life*, September 12 and 25, 1922, Arequipa Collection, Bancroft Library, University of California–Berkeley.

15. Poetry in Arequipa Collection, Bancroft Library, University of California–Berkeley.

16. *Hi-Life*, May 12, 1922, Arequipa Collection, Bancroft Library, University of California–Berkeley.

17. *Hi-Life*, September 25, 1921, Arequipa Collection, Bancroft Library, University of California–Berkeley.

18. *Hi-Life*, May 12, 1922, Arequipa Collection, Bancroft Library, University of California–Berkeley.

19. D'Antonio, *American Nursing*, 43.

CHAPTER 10. PLEASANT DIVERSIONS, UNPLEASANT TREATMENTS

1. Charles L. Minor, "The Psychological Handling of the Tuberculous Patient," *American Review of Tuberculosis* 2 (October 1918): 462.

2. Broussard, *Black San Francisco*, 77.

3. *Oakland Tribune*, December 21, 1919.

4. Arequipa Sanatorium, *Annual Report*, 1922, 21–22.

5. William H. Rosenau, "The Radio and the Tuberculosis Patient," *American Review of Tuberculosis* 5 (May 1926): 475–78.

6. *San Francisco Chronicle*, July 3, 1922.

7. Esmond R. Long, "Artificial Pneumothorax in Tuberculosis," *American Journal of Nursing* 19 (January 1919): 265.

8. *Mountaineer*, September 15, 1931, Arequipa Collection, Bancroft Library, University of California–Berkeley.

CHAPTER 11. YOUR GREATEST WISH WILL BE GRANTED

1. Author interviews with Sarah Brown, Andrew Brown, and Charlotte Brown, 2018; *San Francisco Call*, March 22, 1910; *Harvard Class of 1921: Twenty-Fifth Anniversary Report* (Cambridge, Mass: Class of 1921, 1946), 74; James K. Brown, "Growing Up: Six Early Years, 1931–1936" (unpublished memoir).

2. Author interview with Lois Downey, 1983.

CHAPTER 12. A WORLD WITHIN A WORLD

1. *Mountaineer,* September 15, 1931, Arequipa Collection, Bancroft Library, University of California–Berkeley.

2. United States Census, 1900; *San Francisco Call*, November 10, 1912; Iva M. Miller, "Medical Work in Tientsin," *Woman's Missionary Friend* 1 (January 1917): 4; *San Francisco Chronicle*, September 29, 1922; *San Francisco Chronicle*, January 15, 1930; *San Francisco Chronicle*, November 13, 1932.

3. *Oxnard Press-Courier,* December 21, 1928; *Garrett (Indiana) Clipper*, May 22, 1930; *Business Woman* 7 (August 23, 1930): 1; *San Anselmo Herald*, April 10, 1931; *Los Angeles Times*, March 12, 1933.

4. Ethel Owen correspondence, Arequipa Collection, Bancroft Library, University of California–Berkeley.

5. *Mountaineer,* October 25, 1931, Arequipa Collection, Bancroft Library, University of California–Berkeley.

6. *Petaluma Argus-Courier,* October 17, 1934; *San Rafael Daily Independent Journal*, November 4, 1934.

7. United States Army, Base Hospital 12, World War I and World War II records, 1917–2006, Northwestern University Archives, Chicago; *Lansing State Journal*, May 23, 1917; *Northwestern University Bulletin: The President's Report for 1917–1919* 21 (July 17, 1920): 35–38; Vernon K. Brown, *The Story of Passavant Memorial Hospital, 1865–1972* (Chicago: Northwestern Memorial Hospital, 1976), 57, 92.

8. *Quipa-Tab,* 1935, Arequipa Collection, Bancroft Library, University of California–Berkeley.

9. *Quipa-Tab,* 1935.

10. *San Francisco Chronicle,* February 23, 1931; *San Anselmo Herald*, August 6, 1931; *San Francisco Chronicle*, November 12, 1934; *Sausalito News*, January 18, 1935.

11. *San Francisco Chronicle,* September 7, 1936.

12. *Garrett (Indiana) Clipper,* May 22, 1930.

13. *Santa Ana Register,* June 16, 1936; United States Census, 1940; *Stanford Daily*, November 17, 1944.

14. Arequipa Sanatorium, *Annual Report*, 1915, 12; *Santa Cruz Evening News*, October 5, 1920; Philip King Brown, "Industry's Answer: How a Railroad Safeguards Its Employees in Health and Sickness," *Survey Graphic* (January 1930): 398–401; Philip King Brown, "Organized Medicine's Interest in a Health Insurance Plan for Small Wage Earners," *New England Journal of Medicine* 105 (December 31, 1931): 1–18; Philip King Brown, "The Health Insurance Bills before the Legislature," January

1937, Arequipa Collection, Bancroft Library, University of California–Berkeley; Philip King Brown, "The Majority Report of the Committee on the Costs of Medical Care," *Western Hospital Review* 21 (March 1933): 608–9; Michael Dimmitt, *Ninety Years of Health Insurance Reform Efforts in California* (Sacramento: California Research Bureau, 2007): 9–17.

15. James K. Brown, "Growing Up: 1937–1939."

16. Inge Schaefer Horton, *Early Women Architects of the San Francisco Bay Area: The Lies and Work of Fifty Professionals, 1890–1951* (Jefferson, N.C.: McFarland & Company, 2010), 183–86.

17. James K. Brown, "Growing Up: Six Early Years."

18. *California Medical Association Journal* 53 (December 1940): 287.

19. Stanford University, *Alumni Directory and Ten-Year Book, 1891–1920* (Stanford, Calif: Stanford University, 1921), 423; *San Francisco Chronicle*, November 5, 1930

20. San Francisco city directories.

21. Author interview with Marion Dickey, 1987.

CHAPTER 13. MAGIC BULLETS

1. "Survey of Tuberculosis Hospitals and Sanatoriums in the United States," *Journal of the American Medical Association* 105 (1935): 1915.

2. Author interview with Marion Dickey, 1987.

3. Horton, *Early Women Architects*, 101.

4. Author interview with Rose, 2018.

5. Betty MacDonald, *The Plague and I* (Philadelphia: J. B. Lippincott, 1948), 184–87.

6. Author interview with Lois McMurdo, 1984.

7. Caroline Luce, "The White Plague in the City of Angels," *University of Southern California,* http://scalar.usc.edu/hc/tuberculosis-exhibit/index (accessed December 7, 2018); Ray M. Merrill, Spencer S. Davis, Gordon B. Lindsay, and Elena Khomitch, "Explanations for 20th Century Tuberculosis Decline: How the Public Gets It Wrong," *Journal of Tuberculosis Research* 4 (2016): 111–21; Rene Dubos and Jean Dubos, *The White Plague: Tuberculosis, Man and Society* (Boston: Little, Brown, 1952), 154–56; Sheila M. Rothman, *Living in the Shadow of Death: Tuberculosis and the Social Experience of Illness in American History* (New York: Basic Books, 1994), 247–49.

8. Handwritten note in Arequipa Collection, Bancroft Library, University of California–Berkeley.

9. J. H. Elliott, "Pregnancy and Tuberculosis," *American Review of Tuberculosis* 4 (December 1920): 792–97.

10. American Lung Association, "The History of Christmas Seals," *American Lung Association*, 2018, www.christmasseals.org/history/ (accessed October 1, 2018).

11. Author interview with "Patty," 1984.

CHAPTER 14. DANCING BACK TO BED

1. *San Francisco Chronicle*, June 5, 1993; *Pacific Sun*, June 11, 1993.

2. Letters and affidavits prepared by Roger Kent, 1950–1952, Arequipa Collection, Bancroft Library, University of California–Berkeley.

3. *San Rafael Daily Independent Journal*, August 16, 1951, September 12, 1951, November 14, 1951, December 19, 1951, June 19, 1952.

4. *Life*, March 3, 1952, 20.

5. Author interview with "Bonnie," 1984.

6. *San Rafael Daily Independent Journal*, April 11, 1953; *Auburn (California) Journal*, December 17, 1953.

7. *Sausalito News*, December 3, 1953.

8. *San Rafael Daily Independent Journal*, October 16, 1953.

9. Correspondence, Arequipa Collection, Bancroft Library, University of California–Berkeley.

10. *San Rafael Daily Independent Journal,* December 13, 1955.

11. *San Rafael Daily Independent Journal,* April 9, 1956.

12. *San Rafael Daily Independent Journal,* May 12, 1954, July 1, 1954, July 19, 1954; *Sausalito News*, December 16, 1955.

13. Helen Thompson, "The Evolution of the Nurse Stereotype via Postcards: From Drunk to Saint to Sexpot to Modern Medical Professional," *Smithsonian*, September 24, 2014, https://www.smithsonianmag.com/history/evolution-nurse-stereotype -postcards-drunk-saint-sexpot-modern-medical-professional-180952725/ (accessed December 7, 2018).

14. *San Rafael Daily Independent Journal*, March 14, 1956, April 12, 1957, June 8, 1957.

15. *San Rafael Daily Independent Journal*, June 8, 1957; *Sausalito News*, December 28, 1957.

16. *Bulletin of the Marin County Medical Society* 3 (January 1958): 27.

17. *San Rafael Daily Independent Journal*, June 6, 1960, July 11, 1960.

18. Author interview with Cari Lyn Stanton, 2017.

CHAPTER 15. AFTERLIVES

1. *San Francisco Chronicle*, January 1941; *Rochester (New York) Democrat and Chronicle*, May 1, 1965.

2. San Francisco city directories, 1930–1955; *California Medicine* 84 (March 1956): 220.

3. *Stanford Daily*, November 17, 1944; *Santa Cruz Sentinel*, April 7, 1957, November 22, 1957, April 16, 1958; Scandinavian Airlines System, "Air Passenger Manifest," August 12, 1951, *Ancestry.com*, https://search.ancestry.com/cgi-bin/sse.dll?indiv=1&dbid=60882&h =2049987&tid=&pid=&usePUB=true&_phsrc=bbT1515&_phstart=successSource (accessed January 9, 2019); Trans World Airlines, "Passenger Manifest," September 25, 1956, *Ancestry.com*, https://search.ancestry.com/cgi-bin/sse.dll?indiv=1&dbid =7488&h=3041232987&tid=&pid=&usePUB=true&_phsrc=bbT1516&_phstart =successSource (accessed January 9, 2019); Treasury Department, United States Customs Service, "Passenger List, Crew List," 1960, *Ancestry.com*, https://search .ancestry.com/cgi-bin/sse.dll?indiv=1&dbid=9127&h=189311&tid=&pid=&usePUB =true&_phsrc=bbT1522&_phstart=successSource (accessed January 9, 2019); *Santa Cruz Sentinel*, December 14, 1969.

4. *Salem (Oregon) Statesman Journal*, August 12, 1961; *Sacramento Bee*, April 1, 1946; Ancestry.com, "California, San Francisco Area Funeral Home Records, 1895–1985," *Ancestry.com*, https://search.ancestry.com/cgi-bin/sse.dll?indiv=1&dbid =2118&h=437923&tid=&pid=&usePUB=true&_phsrc=bbT1525&_phstart=success-Source (accessed January 9, 2019).

5. Author interview with Rose, 2018; *San Rafael Independent Journal*, February 2, 1974.

6. *San Anselmo Herald*, February 16, 1945.

7. J. B. Lyon, *Historical Sketches of Franklin County and Its Several Towns* (Albany: J. B. Lyon, 1918), 40–41; *Hartford Courant*, April 3, 1929, May 29, 1938, January 30, 1942, July 1, 1948.

8. State Board of Charities and Corrections, *Tenth Biennial Report of the State Board of Charities and Corrections of the State of California, from July 1, 1920, to June 30, 1922* (Sacramento: State Board of Charities and Corrections, 1923), 72; *Los Angeles Times*, March 29, 1925; *Oakland Tribune*, January 20, 1926; California Department of Public Health, *Weekly Bulletin* (February 5, 1927): 206; United States Census, 1930.

9. U.S. Department of Labor, Immigration Service, "List or Manifest of Alien Passengers for the United States," June 28, 1920, *Ancestry*.com, https://search.ancestry. com/cgi-bin/sse.dll?indiv=1&dbid=6061&h=105960385&tid=&pid=&usePUB =true&_phsrc=bbT1531&_phstart=successSource (accessed January 9, 2019); Alameda County directories, 1920–1929; *Business Women's Herald* 1 (April 21, 1924): 201; United States Census, 1930, 1940; Ancestry.com, "California Death Index, 1940–1997," *Ancestry.com*, https://search.ancestry.com/cgi-bin/sse.dll?indiv=1&dbid =5180&h=3077598&usePUB=true&_phsrc=bbT1540&_phstart=successSource &requr=2550866976735232&ur=0&lang=en-US (accessed January 9, 2019).

10. United States Census, 1930; San Francisco city directories, 1931–1939; "California Death Index."

11. *San Francisco Chronicle*, June 2, 1936; "Great Register of Voters"; *Oakland Tribune*, December 9, 1941; "California Death Index."

12. Northwestern University Archives, Chicago.

13. *The Story of the Hamilton Health Association: Seventeenth Annual Report* (Hamilton, Ont.: Hamilton Health Association, 1921), 13; *San Francisco Chronicle*, February 12, 1935.

14. *San Francisco Chronicle*, July 17, 1920; *Oakland Tribune*, February 2, 1922; *San Francisco Chronicle*, May 27, 1923; *Bulletin of the California Council of Social Work* 6 (August 1923): 2; *Bulletin of the California Council of Social Work* 7 (December 1923): 2, 20; United States Census, 1930, 1940; *San Francisco Chronicle*, October 23, 1941; San Francisco city directories, 1915–1962; author interview with Lois McMurdo, 1984.

15. Ancestry.com, "California, Wills and Probate Records, 1850–1953 for Jeannette Jordan," *Ancestry.com*, https://search.ancestry.com/cgi-bin/sse.dll?indiv=1&dbid =8639&h=1345440&tid=&pid=&usePUB=true&_phsrc=bbT1550&_phstart=suc-cessSource (accessed January 9, 2019); Arequipa Sanatorium, *Annual Report*, 1922, 13.

16. Biographical material, Telegraph Hill Neighborhood Center Archives, San Francisco.

17. Casey, *Henry E. Bothin*, 369–86, passim.

18. Author interview with "Patty"; *San Rafael Independent Journal*, May 20, 2017.

19. Author interview with "Bonnie"; *San Rafael Independent Journal*, February 15, 2004.

20. Author interview with Rose, 2018.

21. *Medford (Oregon) Mail Tribune*, October 10, 1960; *San Rafael Independent Journal*, May 2, 1963; *Sausalito News*, March 26, 1953; author interviews with Andrew Brown, Charlotte Brown, and Sarah Brown.

22. Anema, *Ynes Mexia*, 27–125, passim.

23. Dale, *Frederick Hurten Rhead*, 93–123; Kenneth R. Trapp and Kim Cooper, "Biographies and Company Histories," in Trapp, *The Arts and Crafts Movement in California*, 288–89, 294.

24. Albert Solon to Philip King Brown, 1930, Arequipa Collection, Bancroft Library, University of California–Berkeley.

25. Roorbach, "Art as a Tonic," 346.

BIBLIOGRAPHY

MANUSCRIPT COLLECTIONS AND MATERIALS

American Red Cross records. Commission for France. Hoover Institution. Stanford University.

Arequipa Sanatorium records. Bancroft Library. University of California–Berkeley.

Countway Library of Medicine. Archives and Records Management. Harvard University Medical School.

Frank Norris Collection of Papers and Related Materials. Bancroft Library. University of California–Berkeley.

Gleeson Library. Special Collections. University of California–San Francisco.

Northwestern University Archives.

Philip King Brown papers. Lane Medical Archives. Stanford University Medical Center.

Telegraph Hill Neighborhood Center Archives.

Ynés Mexía papers. Bancroft Library. University of California–Berkeley.

ORAL HISTORY INTERVIEWS

Lois Downey, 1983

"Patty," 1984

"Bonnie," 1984

Phoebe Hearst Brown, 1984

Lois McMurdo, 1984

Marion Dickey, 1987

Cari Lyn Stanton, 2017

Rose, 2018

Andrew Brown, 2018

Charlotte Brown, 2018

Sarah Brown, 2018

BOOKS AND ARTICLES

American Medical Association. *American Medical Directory.* Chicago: American Medical Association, 1921.

Anema, Durlynn. *Ynes Mexia: Botanist and Adventurer.* Greensboro, N.C.: Morgan Reynolds, 2005.

Baizerman, Suzanne, Lynn Downey, and John Toki. *Fired by Ideals: Arequipa Pottery and the Arts & Crafts Movement.* San Francisco: Pomegranate, 2000.

Barker, Malcolm E., ed. *Three Fearful Days: San Francisco Memoirs of the 1906 Earthquake and Fire.* San Francisco: Londonborn, 1988.

Barnes, Harry Lee. "Food Complaints in Sanatoria." *Journal of the Outdoor Life* 25 (January 1928): 10–14.

Baxandall, Rosalyn, Linda Gordon, and Susan Reverby, eds. *America's Working Women: A Documentary History, 1600 to the Present.* New York: Vintage Books, 1976.

Broussard, Albert S. *Black San Francisco: The Struggle for Racial Equality in the West, 1900–1954.* Lawrence: University Press of Kansas, 1993.

Brown, Adelaide. "The History of the Development of Women in Medicine in California." *California and Western Medicine* 23 (May 1925): 579–81.

Brown, Charlotte. "A Thesis on Therapeutic Adjuvants or Minor Medicine." Thesis, Woman's Medical College of Pennsylvania, 1873–74.

———. *The Health of Our Girls.* San Francisco: Woodward & Co., 1896.

Brown, Helen Hillyer. *For My Children and Grandchildren.* San Francisco: Hillside Press, 1986.

———. *The Great San Francisco Fire.* San Francisco: Leo Holub, 1956.

———. "The History of the Arequipa Pottery." Unpublished manuscript, 1914.

Brown, James K. "Growing Up: Six Early Years, 1931–1936." Unpublished manuscript.

———. "Growing Up: 1937–1939." Unpublished manuscript.

Brown, Philip King. "By Six-to-One in California." *Survey Graphic* 27 (November 1938): 609–11.

———. "Eighteen Years' Experience with Ergotherapy." In *Transactions of the Fourteenth Annual Meeting, June 6–8, 1918.* National Tuberculosis Association, 1918.

———. "The Health Insurance Bills before the Legislature," January 1937. Arequipa Collection, Bancroft Library, University of California–Berkeley.

———. "Industry's Answer: How a Railroad Safeguards Its Employees in Health and Sickness." *Survey Graphic* 19 (January 1930): 398–401.

———. "Interesting Comments from Paris." *California State Journal of Medicine* 17 (January 1919): 29.

———. "The Majority Report of the Committee on the Costs of Medical Care." *Western Hospital Review* 21 (March 1933): 608–9.

———. "Medicine's Interest in the Next California Legislature." *California and Western Medicine* 46 (February 1937): 140–41.

———. *The Opening of a Sanatorium for Early Cases of Tuberculosis in Wage-Earning Women.* San Francisco: San Francisco Polyclinic, 1911.

———. "Organized Medicine's Interest in a Health Insurance Plan for Small Wage Earners." *New England Journal of Medicine* 205 (December 31, 1931): 1285–91.

———. "The Outdoor Life in California." *Journal of the Outdoor Life* 5 (March 1908): 45–48.

———. "Tuberculosis Class Work in the San Francisco Polyclinic." *Merchants Association Review* 14 (September 1909): 5–6.

Brown, Vernon K. *The Story of Passavant Memorial Hospital, 1865–1972.* Chicago: Northwestern Memorial Hospital, 1976.

Callen, Anthea. *Angel in the Studio: Women in the Arts and Crafts Movement, 1870–1914.* London: Astragal Books, 1979.

Carrington, Thomas Spees. *Tuberculosis Hospital and Sanatorium Construction.* New York: National Association for the Study and Prevention of Tuberculosis, 1914.

Casey, Michael. *Henry E. Bothin: Philanthropist of Steel.* Nicasio, Calif.: Michael Casey, 2015.

Council on Medical Education and Hospitals. "Survey of Tuberculosis Hospitals and Sanatoriums in the United States." *Journal of the American Medical Association* 105 (December 7, 1935): 1855–1916.

Craddock, Susan. *City of Plagues: Disease, Poverty, and Deviance in San Francisco.* Minneapolis: University of Minnesota Press, 2000.

Dale, Sharon. *Frederick Hurten Rhead: An English Potter in America.* Erie, Pa.: Erie Art Museum, 1986.

Daniels, Douglas Henry. *Pioneer Urbanites: A Social and Cultural History of Black San Francisco.* Philadelphia: Temple University Press, 1980.

D'Antonio, Patricia. *American Nursing: A History of Knowledge, Authority, and the Meaning of Work.* Baltimore: Johns Hopkins University Press, 2010.

Davies, Margery W. *Woman's Place is at the Typewriter: Office Work and Office Workers, 1870–1930.* Philadelphia: Temple University Press, 1982.

Dimmitt, Michael. *Ninety Years of Health Insurance Reform Efforts in California.* Sacramento: California Research Bureau, 2007.

Dinnean, Lawrence. *Les Jeunes: An Account of Some Fin de Siècle San Francisco Authors and Artists.* Berkeley: Friends of the Bancroft Library, 1980.

Dubos, Rene, and Jean Dubos. *The White Plague: Tuberculosis, Man and Society.* Boston: Little, Brown, 1952.

Eichel, Otto R. "Women's Clubs and Tuberculosis." *Journal of the Outdoor Life* 14 (April 1917): 104–6.

Eliassen, Meredith. "The San Francisco Experiment: Female Medical Practitioners Caring for Women and Children, 1875–1935." *Gender Forum* 25 (2009): 31–43.

Evans, Paul. *Art Pottery of the United States.* New York: Feingold and Lewis, 1987.

Fried, Stephen. *Appetite for America: How Visionary Businessman Fred Harvey Built a Railroad Hospitality Empire That Civilized the Wild West.* New York: Random House, 2010.

Genevieve, Sister Rose. "Diet in Tuberculosis." *Journal of the Outdoor Life* 25 (January 1928): 15–17.

Groth, Paul. *Living Downtown: The History of Residential Hotels in the United States.* Berkeley: University of California Press, 1994.

Harris, E. L. *The Shadowmakers: A History of Radiologic Technology.* Albuquerque: American Society of Radiologic Technologists, 1995.

Harris, Henry. *California's Medical Story.* San Francisco: J. W. Stacey, 1932.

Hjalmarson, Birgitta. *Artful Players: Artistic Life in Early San Francisco.* Los Angeles: Balcony Press, 1999.

Hofstadter, Richard. *The Progressive Movement, 1900–1915*. Englewood Cliffs, N.J.: Prentice-Hall, 1963.

Hoover, Jennifer A. Bloom. "Diversional Occupational Therapy in World War I: A Need for Purpose in Occupations." *American Journal of Occupational Therapy* 50 (November/December 1996): 881–85.

Horton, Inge Schaefer. *Early Women Architects of the San Francisco Bay Area: The Lies and Work of Fifty Professionals, 1890–1951*. Jefferson N.C.: McFarland & Company, 2010.

Hotaling, Mary B. *A Rare Romance in Medicine: The Life and Legacy of Edward Livingston Trudeau*. Saranac Lake, N.Y.: Historic Saranac Lake, 2016.

Hutchinson, Woods. "The Health of Working-Women." *Saturday Evening Post* 182 (November 20, 1909): 3–5, 49–50.

Knopf, S. Adolphus. "Woman's Duty in the Combat of Tuberculosis." *Journal of the Outdoor Life* 13 (November 1916): 347–48.

Krafft, Elsie. "The Mental Hygiene Clinic (from the Standpoint of a Social Worker). *Pacific Coast Journal of Nursing* 15 (January 1919): 27–29.

LaMotte, Ellen Newbold. *The Tuberculosis Nurse: Her Function and Her Qualifications*. New York: G. P. Putnam's Sons, 1915.

Lewis, Oscar. *Bay Window Bohemia: An Account of the Brilliant Artistic World of Gaslit San Francisco*. Garden City, N.Y.: Doubleday, 1956.

Long, Esmond R. "Artificial Pneumothorax in Tuberculosis." *American Journal of Nursing* 19 (January 1919): 265–68.

Longstreth, Richard. *On the Edge of the World: Four Architects in San Francisco at the Turn of the Century*. New York: Architectural History Foundation, 1983.

Lyon, J. B. *Historical Sketches of Franklin County and Its Several Towns*. Albany: J. B. Lyon Company, 1918.

MacDonald, Betty. *The Plague and I*. Philadelphia: J. B. Lippincott Company, 1948.

Mentzer, Mary Jones. "Perspective in Diagnosis of Pulmonary Tuberculosis." *Modern Medicine* 2 (December 1920): 813–15.

Merrill, Ray, Spencer S. Davis, Gordon B. Lindsay, and Elena Khomitch. "Explanations for 20th Century Tuberculosis Decline: How the Public Gets It Wrong." *Journal of Tuberculosis Research* 4 (2016): 111–21.

Miller, Iva M. "Medical Work in Tientsin." *Woman's Missionary Friend* 1 (January 1917): 3–8.

Minor, Charles L. "The Psychological Handling of the Tuberculous Patient." *American Review of Tuberculosis* 2 (October 1918): 459–69.

Mitchell, Pryce. *Deep Water: The Autobiography of a Sea Captain*. Boston: Little, Brown, 1933.

Morantz-Sanchez, Regina Markell. *Sympathy and Science: Women Physicians in American Medicine*. New York: Oxford, 1985.

Morgan, Shirley. "Well Diary . . . I Have Tuberculosis: Researching a Teenager's 1918 Sanatorium Experience." Unpublished manuscript, 2014.

National Association for the Study and Prevention of Tuberculosis. *A Tuberculosis Directory: A List of Institutions, Associations and Other Agencies Dealing with*

Tuberculosis in the United States and Canada. New York: National Association for the Study and Prevention of Tuberculosis, 1911.

————. *A Tuberculosis Directory: A List of Institutions, Associations and Other Agencies Dealing with Tuberculosis in the United States and Canada*. New York: National Association for the Study and Prevention of Tuberculosis, 1919.

Ott, Katherine. *Fevered Lives: Tuberculosis in American Culture since 1870*. Cambridge: Harvard University Press, 1996.

Report of the Health Officer of the City and County of San Francisco for the Fiscal Year Ending June 30, 1875. San Francisco: Spaulding and Barto, Steam Book and Job Printers, 1875.

Richardson, Heather Cox. *West from Appomattox: The Reconstruction of America after the Civil War*. New Haven, Conn.: Yale University Press, 2007.

Robinson, Judith. *The Hearsts: An American Dynasty*. New York: Avon Books, 1991.

Rosenau, William H. "The Radio and the Tuberculosis Patient." *American Review of Tuberculosis* 5 (May 1926): 475–78.

Rothhammer, Amilu S. "A Lofty Mountain to Scale: A Tale of Perseverance." *Archives of Surgery Journal* 136 (May 2001): 499–504.

Rothman, Sheila M. *Living in the Shadow of Death: Tuberculosis and the Social Experience of Illness in American History*. New York: Basic Books, 1994.

Sachs, Theodore B. "The Tuberculosis Nurse." *American Journal of Nursing* (May 1908): 597–98.

Sagar, William, and Brian Sagar. *Fairfax: Images of America*. Charleston: Arcadia Publishing, 2005.

San Francisco Blue Book. San Francisco: Charles C. Hoag, 1909.

San Francisco Polyclinic. *Annual Report*. San Francisco: San Francisco Polyclinic, 1892.

Sklar, Kathryn Kish. "The 'Quickened Conscience': Women's Voluntarism and the State, 1890–1920." *Institute for Philosophy and Public Policy Quarterly* 18 (1998): 27–33.

Solberg, Gunnard. *Hill Farm and Arequipa*. Fairfax, Calif.: Fairfax Historical Society, 1997.

Taylor, Robert. *Saranac: America's Magic Mountain*. Boston: Houghton, Mifflin 1986.

Tentler, Leslie Woodcock. *Wage Earning Women: Industrial Work and Family Life in the United States, 1900–1930*. New York: Oxford, 1979.

"The Tuberculosis Convalescent: After the Sanitarium or Preliminary Rest Cure at Home—What Next." *Journal of the Outdoor Life* 6 (May 1909): 123–26.

Thelander, H. E. "Children's Hospital of San Francisco." *Medical Woman's Journal* (July 1934): 184–98.

Trapp, Kenneth R., ed. *The Arts and Crafts Movement in California: Living the Good Life*. Oakland, Calif.: Oakland Museum, 1993.

Trudeau, Edward Livingston. "The Part of Women in Tuberculosis Work." *Journal of the Outdoor Life* 6 (April 1909): 91–92.

Tygiel, Jules. *Workingmen in San Francisco, 1880–1901*. New York: Garland, 1992.

Walker's Manual of California Securities and Directory of Directors. San Francisco: H. D. Walker, 1910.

Wertheimer, Barbara Mayer. *We Were There: The Story of Working Women in America.*
    New York: Pantheon Books, 1977.
White, Mary L. "The Training School for Nurses in San Francisco." *Overland Monthly
    and Out West Magazine* 9 (February 1887): 123–28.
"Women Pay Their Way while Under Treatment." *Modern Hospital* 2 (March 1914):
    178–79.

INDEX

Page numbers in *italics* indicate illustrations.

Printed in the USA
CPSIA information can be obtained
at www.ICGtesting.com
CBHW031404210524
8886CB00001B/17